# *BEHIND THE SCENES*
# *IN*
# *NURSING*

YVONNE SAM

# *Behind the Scenes*
## *in*
## *Nursing*

**ISBN: 978-1-990420-17-7**

Published by: Labworks Publishing Inc.
www.labworkspublishing.com
labworkspublishing@gmail.com

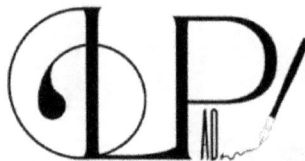

LABWORKS PUBLISHING AD

# DEDICATION

This nursing memoir is dedicated to you, Mom and Dad, with all my love and gratitude. Thank you for never accepting less than an A, and for making me the wonderful human being that I have become. This completed work is truly yours.

Also to all the many nurses I have encountered in my life, and those I will never meet. Nevertheless, we remain sisters and brothers bonded in service.

# ACKNOWLEDGEMENTS

I am thankful for the gifts that God the Father has bestowed on me -- the strength that keeps me standing, the grace that passes all understanding, and the realization that through Him all things are possible.

I thank every nursing instructor, every nursing student, every nurse, every doctor, every medical student with whom I have worked. I thank every patient whom I have encountered during my career, who unknowingly taught me what the textbooks failed to do.

To my many mentors, far and near, thanks for your guidance.

Finally, I am eternally grateful to my sons Wilbert and Christopher, who not only served as my tech savvy agents, but who also helped in keeping me mentally balanced and focused throughout, at times an overwhelming task for both them and me. I deeply appreciate their understanding and love. I am most proud of them, as they are of me.

# CONTENTS

# PROLOGUE

> "I attribute my success to this: I never gave or took an excuse."
> — *Florence Nightingale*

This is the story of my life-long education as a nurse. The events and encounters related in this memoir span three continents. They take place in several hospitals and healthcare facilities, and are not limited to a nursing speciality. I include my experiences as a student nurse, midwife, psychiatric nurse and finally a Head Nurse. I reveal what goes on behind bedside curtains, in cubicles, on the Unit, on Admission and Assessment Units, Labor & Delivery rooms, in medication rooms and staff lounges.

Within these pages, I have attempted to explain the challenges nurses face working within a healthcare system, which sometimes fail those who partake and those who provide. In pointing out perceived weaknesses and flaws, I respectfully offer my own ideas for practical improvements and resolutions. Admittedly, this is my opportunity to atone for the occasions when I could have spoken up, but I did not. It is now plainly obvious that my reticence, besides a natural tendency to mind my own business, was due to fear of reprisal, ignorance of accepted norms and youthful inexperience.

A nurse can make a difference between life and death, a concept that can never be overstated. They serve as a voice for the marginalized, and comfort for the suffering. The great majority of nurses are faithful to their creed, but when the few fail in that effort or commitment, blame should not be placed but rather recognition of the need for improvement so that they can continue in the immeasurable good to which these "angels of mercy" devote so much of their lives.

# CHAPTER 1
# ANSWERED PRAYERS

"It's not the traveling that takes courage...It's leaving home"
— *Scott Westerfield*

I was born in Georgetown, Guyana, officially the Cooperative Republic of Guyana, the only English- speaking country on the northern mainland of South America, the second child of ten siblings, born to George a hard- working night watchman and his self-employed, work- from -home wife Harriet. Despite having so many siblings, my early years were spent in modest, yet comfortable surroundings. As I recall my parents were unfalteringly inspired by the belief that their collective sacrifices would ensure that all their children would receive, as my mother so resolutely put it, "a sound primary and a concrete secondary education".

My father earned his living as a night watchman, employed by (Radio Demerara) the sole radio broadcasting station in the country; while my mother sold homemade pastries and jams to the locals, even serving as a supplier for certain well- known grocery stores in the city. My parents regularly reminded my siblings and me of the importance of education as being the key to a successful future. In the spirit of true parental love and devotion they had pledged to stand on guard for us all, a responsibility that demonstrably they were not taking lightly. In the neighbourhood, our home was the only one with children attending secondary school, and top ones to boot.

My two younger brothers George Jnr. and Raphael attended Queens College, an all-boys secondary school, notably the most prestigious educational institution in the history of the country. From time to time my parents would brag about my brothers' presence at the top rated institution of higher learning, as if my attendance at another equally rated private, secondary school, was not of the same significance. Despite this seeming parental disinterest, I was nevertheless maintaining equally good grades. My parents had made it absolutely that mediocrity in academic studies would not be tolerated.

Following graduation from secondary school with a College of Preceptors Certificate, General Certificate of Education, Ordinary and Advanced Level I taught for a brief period at a rural elementary school, following which I entered the Civil Service as a junior clerk, in the Final Accounts Section, Ministry of Finance. As the youngest member of the clerical staff, I took advantage of the time spent in the company of the older and senior personnel. Admittedly, along with my prior working environment it assisted in shaping my burgeoning view of the world.

I still recall, and will always treasure the nuggets of wisdom, and gems of advice that were frequently imparted to me by the older and seemingly wiser staff. Some of these gems would later serve as my personal credo.

One day, without any prior warning, I began experiencing auditory incursions, coupled with repeated swirling thoughts, all culminating in an inexplicable urge to travel. Initially, this unheralded auditory phenomenon was almost inaudible, however, as the days progressed this quickly changed, becoming louder and more persistent. Thoughts of foreign lands and faraway places ravaged my thoughts, creating a sense of quasi-uneasiness. I was feeling the urge to leave my country in search of a better life and exciting prospects. Battling the growing mental restlessness, and swirling thoughts caused me to act strangely at times. In the absence of any coercion or persuasion England became the country of choice for my intended migration.

Setting my thoughts in motion, and in the absence of any form of parental invocation or consultation, I completed and forwarded three applications for admission to nurse training schools in England. Such a course of action, did very little however, to quieten the inner excitement that constantly played havoc with my mind.

The manner in which I had dealt with my parents regarding the nursing application, made me quite uneasy. Neither my mother nor my father had done anything to warrant estrangement from my plans, so returning home from work, one evening I decided that I would come clean and disclose to my mother what I had done regarding the sending of the nursing school applications. Immediately, my thoughts centered on her likely reactions: Would she think that I had taken leave of my senses? or Would I be scolded for failing to seek parental counsel before engaging in such an activity? At suppertime I sat at the dinner table, slowly formulating intelligible sentences, while gradually mustering the courage to speak. Prior to allowing the first word to leave my lips, I carefully scrutinized my mother's face. Her usual calm demeanor was evident, and this served to put my mind at ease.

On completion of my announcement, I remained silent, strangely fearing an unexpected outburst from my mother, or at worst swift admonishment in the presence of my siblings. Instead, my mother slowly reached for my hand, and drew me closer to her. She then looked directly into my face, with a smile that lit up her entire face, and in a slightly cracking voice she said, "I am so proud of you". What a feeling of relief slowly enshrouded me, having feared the worst!

Almost six weeks to the date of transmission of the nursing school application, as I approached the front door of our residence, I could hear sounds of laughter, interspersed with off-key singing all coming from inside the house. Nervously, I opened the door, and was greeted by my Mother gazing upwards, with hands raised as if giving praise and reverence to the Almighty, while my other siblings looked on as if a performance was about to begin, and one they did not want to miss.

All eyes were fixed on my mother, following her every move. Slowly but purposefully my mother advanced towards me, while I was still attempting to close the door, her hands clutching what appeared to be a letter protruding from a half-opened envelope, and began to speak in a strangely hurried tone. Initially, I did not understand what she was saying, until I heard the words nursing school, acceptance, and looking forward among the partially-completed sentences. The prize possession that remained firmly clutched in her hands proved to be my acceptance letter from a psychiatric hospital in Essex, England.

The loud noise and incessant chatter that followed the announcement of my acceptance into nursing school, awakened Dad from his pre-work slumber, and without any note of inquiry he hastily requested a lowering of voices, further reminding all present that he needed to rest in preparation for work later. Seemingly misunderstanding Dad's request for tranquility, Mom lost no time in stating the reason behind the merriment, and in a clearly sleepy voice and puzzled look 'he uttered, "I am very proud of you, my dear", quickly closing the bedroom door in order to drown out the din and resume sleeping.

The acceptance letter brought with it a plethora of emotions, and in its wake an entirely new and different meaning for the word 'proud'. I was beginning to feel somewhat apart from my other siblings. Compounding the onset of this inexplicable strange feeling of pride and elation, was an unfamiliar disquietude. Slowly, the atmosphere at home began to take on a new form, as my siblings reluctantly came to the realization of what was beginning to play out before their very eyes, and outside of their control-----that one day soon I would be leaving for England, a country that they knew nothing of, except what had been read in books, the newspapers or heard on the radio. Each time that any mention or reference was made of my leaving, a part of "me" tore inside, immediately forcing me to question myself as to whether or not I had made the right decision to leave my native country and parental security. In beginning nurse training, I would be starting a life far away from my parents and siblings.

Besides my siblings and my parents nothing else in my immediate environment now held any significance for me. I felt as if I were straddling two worlds. All that I had read about London—the double decker busses, the pigeons that frequented and resided in Trafalgar Square, the infamous London Tower— became anticipated realities.

At work my once cheerful countenance was replaced by the occasional pensive look, and half-hearted smile. Conversations became brief, and of a more serious nature. Coworkers made me the butt of their jokes, being overheard daily proffering a plethora of reasons for my altered demeanor, that ran the gamut from the humorously sublime to the insanely ridiculous. Despite the existing shared level of friendship, my impending migration to England remained a well-guarded secret. There was absolutely no discussion, inference or allusion whatsoever, regarding the reality that I would soon be classified as a former employee.

No explanation was ever supplied for my sudden change in behavior and temperament, preferring to wait until travel plans were fully finalized. In an effort to ensure that my imminent departure remained a well-kept secret, I tearfully asked my mother not to put my name on the prayer list at church. In addition to not wanting anyone to be aware of my migratory plans, there was also the desire to not be the object of sympathy or misguided concern, should plans not materialize. Unlike Florence Nightingale, the famed Lady with the Lamp, it was not a call from God that made me choose nursing as a career, but instead the care and affection that the nurses gave my six month old sister, as she lay dying in the Pediatric ward of the local hospital from a recent outbreak of poliomyelitis that had ravaged our island.

I can still hear the crackling sounds that accompanied each waning respiration, and see the lessening of the rise and fall of her tiny chest wall, as I stood by her cot, my head resting on the shoulder of my grieving mother.

Additionally, I still recall seeing the loving, caring way in which the nurse cradled my sister Jacqueline's limp body after she had ceased breathing. A few minutes later a doctor arrived on the scene (seemingly having been summoned by the nurse), and painstakingly began examining my sister, finally pronouncing death, and offering his condolences to my mother, whose face now bore an extremely sad appearance. I looked on tearfully as my mother cradled my deceased sister in her arms, ran her fingers through her hair, staring lovingly and longingly into her pale face, as if not fully understanding what she had just been told by the doctor.

With the love, and care that only a parent can demonstrate towards their own, my mother gently laid my sister back in her crib, planting a kiss on her cheek before covering her face with the blanket. My mother gently clasped my hand, beckoning that it was time to leave. A cacophony of baby cries seemed to join us in our grief, as we slowly walked towards the exit of the Pediatric Unit. It was at this point that I firmly resolved that no matter what I wanted to become a nurse, like the ones who had just demonstrated such loving care towards a dead infant.

# MIGRATION

One mid-September morning, British Airways Flight BA 692 with stops in Trinidad, Barbados, Antigua, Bermuda and finally Heathrow Airport in London, departed from Atkinson Airport in Georgetown, Guyana, carrying among its passengers an individual, mentally and academically but not emotionally ready to embark on a career in nursing.

Eleven hours prior to my arrival in fog-filled London I had said good-bye to my parents, siblings, relatives, friends, neighbours, well-wishers, my childhood home and even my native land. A lot was riding on my shoulders. I boarded the plane somewhat happy, albeit pensive. For as it slowly taxied along the runaway, the parting words of my maternal aunt, "Study hard and make us proud" kept ringing in my ears. My parents in displayed consensus had uttered a similar entreaty earlier on, "Do not be a fool, follow rules, and remember books not boys".

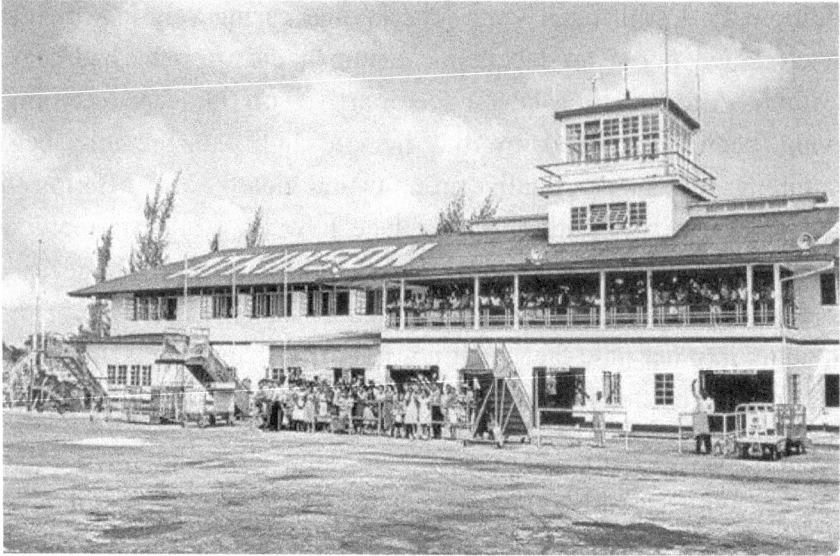

*Atkinson Airport, Georgetown, Guyana.*

*Immigrant Visa (Great Britain)*

With my seat belt securely fastened and the great iron bird slowly gaining altitude towards the welcoming blue skies, the feeling that should I ever veer off course during my educational sojourn Aunt Adina, and my parents would suddenly appear from nowhere, ready to institute their antiquated brand of discipline, brought a smile to my face.

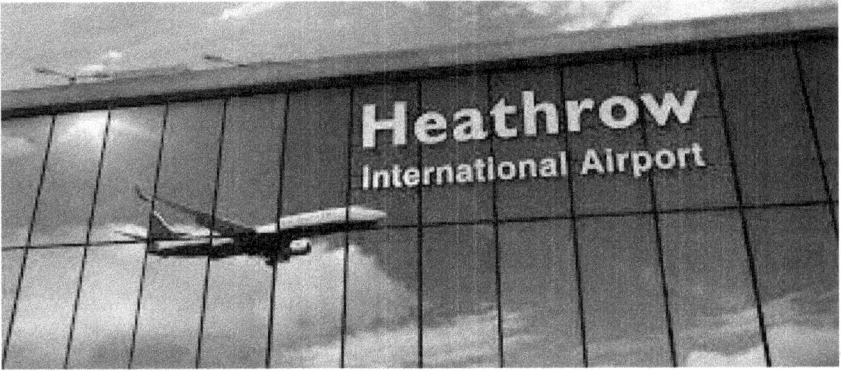

*Heathrow Airport, Hounslow, Middlesex*

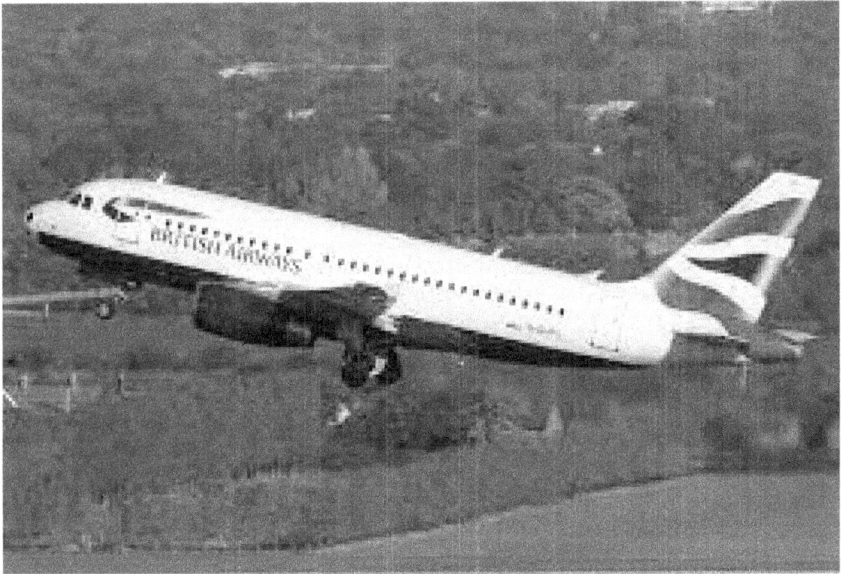

*British Airways*

After being subjected to a barrage of questions by the Immigration officials, and being granted my visa to reside and study in England I now headed towards the clearly identified ARRIVALS LOUNGE, where I quickly became overwhelmed and consumed by the hustle and bustle of the swirling crowd. Never, in my life had I seen so many people in one place at any given time. I had to stop and take it all in, reminding myself that I was now in a foreign country, miles away from my native land.

Suddenly over the public address system I heard my name being announced, requesting that I report to the Information Desk in the arrivals section. "I have suddenly become important", I thought.

On responding to being summoned, after speaking with the bespectacled uniformed officer, I was immediately shown to the door, where a cab was waiting to take me to my new home and training school, courtesy of my new employer. After giving my two suitcases to the driver, I boarded the cab, which quickly exited the airport, joining the busy flow of London's mid-morning traffic. Bobbies with their tall plumed helmets, the roundabouts, double decker-busses and quaint red telephone booths, all of which I had only seen in pictures now captured my full and immediate attention. The rigor of the long transatlantic flight was also beginning to take its toll, as from time to time I found myself nodding off. After the initial greeting, the cab driver had not uttered an additional word, and I found myself succumbing to a descending feeling of sadness. England would be my home for the next three years, while I pursued my nursing career—a lifetime of sorts? a prison sentence? a banishment? a self- inflicted punishment? Would I become old and gray before I ever saw my parents and siblings again?

When I finally reached my destination, I was awakened by the rather rapid opening of the cab door, and a slightly austere middle-aged woman offering her hand in greeting. She introduced herself as the Home Warden, a term I had never heard before, and at this point made no effort to have it explained. As I followed her down the cobblestoned path leading to the building that I would be calling "home", I became startlingly aware of the crisp unfamiliar autumn air, and the fallen leaves that lay like a blanket on the ground. On arriving at the front door of the building, she opened the door and ushered me in, then followed slowly closing the door behind her, as if not wanting to make any noise. She then handed me a booklet atop of which lay a set of keys, and in a distinctly authoritative tone of voice she once again welcomed me to London, informed me of my room number and that the booklet contained pertinent information regarding time, date and location of nursing class commencement and above all the expected code of conduct.

Through the window I could see the Home Warden leaving, as her figure gradually disappeared behind the brick buildings, and turning my gaze inwards I noticed my two suitcases stacked in a corner at the other end of the room. Externally, they appeared none the worse for the long journey, and the likely tossing and tumbling to which they must have been subjected to once separated from me. I slowly opened my room door, taking in all that lay before me, even a sink.

On the bed, covered in plastic was a package containing what would eventually be my uniform package --- a blue and white striped dress with a stiff white collar, starched white apron, a white corded belt, (the color changed every year until you are qualified), a pleated circular piece of white material, which when properly folded and pinned would form the nursing cap, and a cape.

Earrings were not allowed, neither were rings, wristwatches or necklaces. Every nurse had to have a fob watch. My own shoes with laces and rubber soles and white stockings would complete the outfit. The hospital was responsible for laundering our uniforms.

I gradually lowered my travel-worn body on to the only seating accommodation in the room ----, a small Victorian type chair whose appearance remained true to its era. What a relief I felt! My mother had completed the packing of my suitcases, since on more than one occasion; I had openly displayed a lack of emotional courage necessary for the completion of such a simple task. Plainly stated and acceptably truthful, I was coping with packing and grieving all at the same time. I brought my suitcases into the room, and as I slowly unpacked, my Bible became partly visible from beneath some garments, being placed there by my mother in stark intimation of what I should daily do, and whom I should remember and call upon when necessary.

Back home the Holy Bible defined our lives and that of my parents in levees of quoted scriptures. There were Biblical allusions for every occasion. My mother possessed an encyclopedic knowledge of the Bible, and was capable of delivering projectiles of opprobrium, showers of admiration and barrages of reproof all couched in appropriate biblical language and terminology. I continued the task at hand to its full completion of almost an hour's duration, pausing for about 20 minutes to consume a small snack delivered to my room, with the sender identified by a small card with the words "Welcome Committee" written on the inside. As my body began to positively respond to the call of Morpheus, I failed to fully take in the room, and all it had to offer beyond the cupboard where I had just hung my unpacked garments, and the sink that immediately caught my attention on first entering the room.

Historically, pre-registration nurse education in Great Britain was hospital based, modelled on an apprenticeship system with schools of nursing attached to large acute hospitals.

Training was mostly hands-on, and ward-based, with interspersed blocks of time spent outside the clinical environment for academic study periods. Lectures were delivered by Nurse Tutors and Medical Consultants (the great majority of doctors were male). Nurse training was of three years duration, leading to State Registration (after successful completion of a final written and practical exam). Student nurses were the main workforce in hospitals, worked like dogs, being paid a mere pittance and were primarily based on the wards. Blocks of time were spent outside the clinical environment in school, for academic study periods.

No student nurse was allowed to marry, and pregnancy meant instant dismissal. In the first year of training, all nursing students were required to live in the nursing quarters, situated on the hospital grounds. This arrangement based on the presumption that this was necessary because a 7-day 24 hour shift roster meant that nurses worked all hours. Added to this was Florence Nightingale's philosophy that the respectability and morality of nurses had to be protected at all costs. Hospitals Administration took their responsibility seriously and believed that there was a moral imperative to protect the respectability of the young single female nurses in their charge. The large number of nurses who were forced to reside in the nurses quarters did so under the watchful eye and bull-dog determination of the Home Sister, constantly on the look-out for those evil " boyfriends and male doctors".

Moreover, Matron was still very much a figure to fear and to be respected by the nursing staff. Her word was law and nurses were only allowed to speak to her or Sister when they were addressed. As for speaking to the doctors, this was not permitted for ordinary nurses unless expressly instructed to do so. Nurses now worked a 42-hour week having previously been reduced from a 48 hour week. The hours were dire, often 10 days on and four off, and nights were 7 on and 7 off. Nurses were discouraged from wearing their uniforms outside of the hospital for reasons of hygiene.

# CHAPTER 2
# ROOKIE

"I can't go back to yesterday, because I was a different person then."
— *Lewis Carroll*

The six weeks of Preliminary Training School went by quickly, almost as if it was over before it had even begun. In school we were taught ethics, about feeding, bed bathing, giving and taking a bedpan or urinal from a male or female patient, dressings, and how to make a hospital bed properly including the mitred corners. There were two practical rooms in the classroom, which were laid out like mini wards. It was here as nurses in training, that we took turns in being the patient, lying in bed, being washed, turned and questioned. Male nurses were only permitted to work on Male Wards, while female nurses could work on either.

The memory of my first day on the ward is still fresh in my mind. Anxiety, apprehension, and nostalgia had kept me awake at times during the night, despite availing myself of a known home- type sleep inducer—hot Ovaltine.

On being suddenly awakened by the bell at 6.00 a.m. I hastily jumped to my feet prepared to shower, dress, eat breakfast and arrive on time on the ward. This was a red letter day of sorts for me—my first full day of contact with the patients. I was assigned to start duty on DOVECOTE WARD, a 40 bed male and female Geriatric Unit.

Dressed in my nurse's uniform, black shoes, white stockings, heavily – starched white apron and white cap, I felt like a picture perfect representative for nurses and nursing wear, as I made my entry on the ward. Following a short introduction by the Ward Sister, to the entire staff, including the kitchen maid and cleaner, I was then handed over to Bridgette, the Staff Nurse who would be responsible for my learning experience during the six week stay on the ward. Reintroduction to my mentor nurse was followed by direct inquiry as to my level of nursing experience.

I soon learned that Monday was the scheduled bath day for all the patients on the ward, and that I would be assisting with the pre- and post-preparation. "Just my luck", I thought. The patients to be bathed were brought to the bath area by the nursing auxiliaries, one at a time, where they quietly sat on a bench, each with a bundle of clothes, awaiting their turn to be called by the staff who would be taking care of their showering.

I was soon caught up in the hustle and bustle around me---patients in various stages of being dressed, some being dried, and others being taken back to the lounge all the while wondering about my capability to handle the tasks that now lay before my very eyes. A light touch on my shoulder brought me startlingly back to reality, and on turning around I came face to face with Bridgette who immediately placed two face cloths into my partly outstretched hands. She quickly explained that one face cloth was solely for the face, hands and all other areas above the waist, and the other was for bottoms, naughty bits and all other spaces and places. I made a quick mental note of all that she had said, and found it strange that I was not asked if I fully understood the directives. Was she of the belief that the information was far too simple to be misunderstood even by a novice such as me?

Thereupon, she strode off, beckoning me to join her. She calmly announced to an elderly bespectacled gentleman sitting on the bench, that I would be the nurse responsible for giving him his bath. His face shone radiantly as she continued speaking, giving him my name, and losing no time in adding the fact that I was a new nurse in training. Even after hearing the last remark, a smile still remained on his face, a reassuring sign that certainly did a lot in bolstering my courage. Under the watchful eyes of my mentor Bridgette I nervously completed the bath, taking more time than was anticipated, partly due to my determination not to make mistakes, while mentally trying to ace the places for the face cloth usage. When I had finished bathing and showering the patient, paying careful attention to the trouble spots learnt in nursing school especially between the toes, groin area and the folds and creases, I assisted him in getting dressed. So far, Bridgette had uttered no comment, silence which I interpreted as meaning that expectations had been met.

It was the daily routine for each patient to be fully dressed and seated in the dining room at mealtimes. Only bedtime snacks and night beverages, tea, coffee, Horlicks, Bournvita etc. were served to the patient while in bed. Breakfast was usually a substantial fare consisting of fried or grilled tomatoes, bacon, sausages, fried or poached eggs, baked beans, kippers or herrings, buttered toast and as much tea as the patient could drink. Coffee failed to make the beverage list, and was never requested. The meals were delivered to the ward in heated trolleys well in advance of the scheduled meal time.

As a junior nurse you started with the cleaning. Cleaning meant water in a bowl, soap suds, with a cloth and a trolley. The bedside locker of each patient had to be wiped down, rubbish removed and ashtray emptied. Yes, patients were allowed to smoke in bed. Once the lockers were all cleaned, the trolley was then cleaned for the next task at hand. Retrospectively, the sluice could also be considered a ward, for not only was it a constant hive of activity, but also the place where the time spent by a junior nurse, was equal if not more, to that of the ward. Flowers were removed from the ward overnight and placed in the sluice, water changed in each vase and returned to the respective owners in the morning.

After coffee break it was back into the sluice, for the cleaning and sterilizing of bedpans, urinals, vomit bowls and wash basins. The sterilizer had the appearance of a deep chest freezer. It had to be filled with water, switched on and allowed to boil away for a fixed period of time. During the training session, no instruction or information was given regarding how to operate the sterilizer, one of which was on every ward.

I left the Geriatric ward and went next to the medical ward, where a scary looking Sister was in charge. You did as you were told and never asked too many questions. The main objective was to perform satisfactorily, be caring to and careful with the patients, and learn as much as you could. As I progressed in my training, I was often left in Charge of the ward at nights with a junior student nurse, relying on the night sister or nursing officers to help with the Controlled Drugs, which were locked in the DDA (Dangerous Drug Act) cupboard. During the night the Nursing officer would come around the various wards and ask for a bedside update on all the patients.

After eighteen months of training, nursing students sat an examination called the Preliminary Exam. This exam had to be passed in order to continue nurse training. After three years there would be a final exam for qualification as a Registered Nurse.

The latter part of my second year in training, found me in the Theatre (Operating Room) for a six week sojourn. Initially, I was grossly petrified on being made aware of such a placement. I was called upon to transport labelled specimens of body parts to the laboratory. My memory vividly recalls being asked to lift a recently-amputated leg on to a trolley and deliver it to a specifically identified room in the basement of the hospital. Was there a reason underlying my being chosen for such a task?

To proclaim that the three years of nurse training went by quickly, would be in part stretching the truth to its utter maximum. Without any intended air of deception, there were innumerable periods when florid thoughts of absconding, going AWOL, or being declared mentally incompetent crept into my mind. Concerned thoughts regarding my parents and siblings, and if they were missing me as much as I was missing them, daily occupied each and every wakeful moment.

The brutally harsh British winters only served to strengthen my resolve to be successful in my training, and all that I did. The patients acted as another incentive, as most of them had become intrigued not only with the geographical location of my homeland, but also with the size of my family and the fact that we all dwelt under the same roof. They viewed leaving my homeland and journeying so far abroad to pursue nursing studies as a brave move worthy of commendation especially on account of my age, as I was still a teenager. At times I felt that such behavior could be attributed to unrecognized insanity.

Nevertheless, I was overjoyed, to say the least, when my three years of training finally came to an end, followed swiftly by the completion of my Final Nursing Examination. Nursing State Registration was now within my grasp. Once the examination results were made available and my success confirmed, I could not wait to share the good news with my parents. As I picked up the telephone, nervously dialing the well-known number, I kept mentally picturing how my Dad would not only brag about my success, but also how the brains came from his side of the family. How I wish that I could have been there, or my parents able to be here, or at best not so far away! Sadly, I had to settle for a telephone call.

When I made the telephone call, my parents were away from the home. Their absence, although somewhat disappointing, only served to heighten my sense of elation. My father, true to form, ensured that the immediate neighborhood was present when later he made the return call to congratulate me on my success. "You have done us both proud, as well as the community", he repeated several times. In the background I could hear the incessant chattering of the neighbors, interspersed with occasional "Congrats" and the barking of dogs, as if they too were pleased with my success.

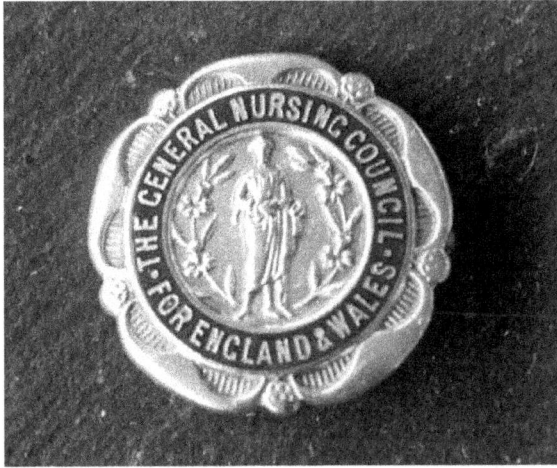

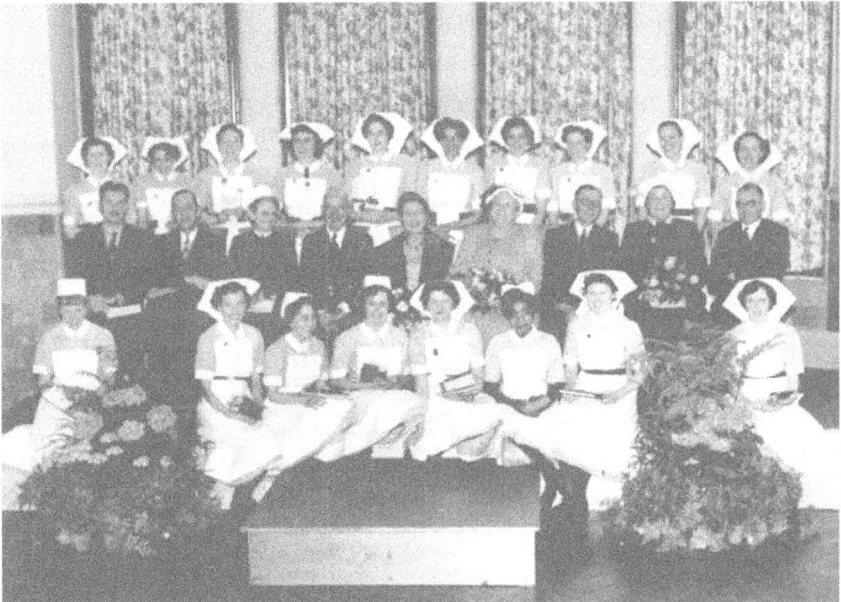

*The author \*back row\* (sixth from left) at graduation*

With my State Registered Nursing Certification now proudly added to my list of achievements, coupled with the relief of having lived up to the expectations of my parents, relatives, and even the matron of the hospital, one would assume that I would take a rest from studies.

In fact, the State Nursing Certification only served to bolster my determination to seek further qualifications. The taste of success was sweet and lingering, and I wanted much more.

I now held the position of Staff Nurse, part of the senior personnel on the ward, a clear transition from sheep to shepherd. With this senior position and title came the responsibility of training the new nursing students arriving on the ward. Strangely enough, three years previously I had been in their shoes, walking somewhat uncomfortably at times. Nevertheless, I now knew how it felt, and I was prepared to dedicate myself to producing quality nurses of the future. Although I thoroughly enjoyed doing what I liked best-----caring for the patients, somehow or other being just a Registered Nurse felt like an unfinished paint job. I had only applied the primer, not even a proper base coat, and the true luster appeared to be lacking. One certificate was certainly not adequate, especially if I wanted to advance further in my career. I was qualified, yet still not satisfied. I wanted more, and I knew that this was just the beginning.

# CHAPTER 3
# MIDWIVES AND PSYCHIATRISTS

"Midwives are there when the first breath is taken, and psychiatrists are there when the mind seems forsaken"

— *Anonymous*

Ten months later, I was once again cast in the student's role— beginning Part 1 of the required training towards becoming a midwife. I was accepted into the Part 1 Midwifery training at Sorrento Maternity Hospital in Birmingham, England. This time however, I entered the Preliminary Training Session or PTS as it was oftentimes referred to, with the confidence of a celebrated boxer, ready for whichever opponent came my way. From time to time I paused to reflect on my personal transformation in just three years. I was conscious of a personal change, although I could not specifically pinpoint the causal factor. Nevertheless, I fully submerged myself into my new training course, literally soaking up in a sponge-like manner, all that was being taught and all that there was to learn. I was determined to claim success once again.

Midwifery training consisted of two parts – the first in hospital and the second in the district. Only with both parts successfully completed, could a midwife become qualified to take on the role of a district midwife. By virtue of the training and practice, midwives became competent and confident to care not only for uncomplicated cases but also to manage, single-handedly, situations that today could make modern hospital midwives reach for the emergency buzzer. In an era before scanning, to a certain extent, every labour could be deemed a journey into the unknown. In Britain midwives are capable of delivering breech babies, twins, premature babies, and those with congenital abnormalities. They are also allowed to administer nitrous oxide for pain relief. They did not carry out any post-delivery suturing, but nevertheless prided themselves on having an intact perineum after birthing a baby.

The Flying Squad was called for obstetric emergencies. This airborne service was provided by local hospitals and consisted of a doctor, midwife, anesthetist, and equipment to manage transfusions and other emergencies at home. During midwifery training the confidence to work alone and to manage complex cases was instilled in pupil midwives.

The pain of childbirth has a way of stripping away the trivial and unimportant, and bringing to the surface what really matters—a healthy newborn. With each delivery, I witnessed or assisted, coupled with the smiles of the mother and sometimes awe-struck father, my training was made more worthwhile. Each delivery was different in its own way, and each one not only bolstered my level of confidence, but also served as a catalyst for improvement for the next delivery. I was enjoying this aspect of nursing far more than the training as a general nurse. With each delivery I felt as if I was a great part of something so much bigger than myself, but then again so much more meaningful and rewarding. As I vicariously went through the stages of labour with each of the patients assigned to my care, I can now describe the process as a marathon of tribulation and consequent triumph, and I have never failed to marvel at each mother's uniform embrace of her baby at the end of it all.

Midwifery training also helped to heighten my level of spiritual awareness, for with each witnessed or assisted birth, it seemed that the Heavenly Father had created females with an uncanny ability to forget pain-- or following delivery did a chemical agent enter the cranial system totally erasing the ordeal they had just underwent?

I whizzed through my initial six months of training, and successfully attained Part I of the State Midwifery Certification. Both the tutors and the Ward –based teacher midwives confessed that never for a moment were they doubtful of my ability to succeed. However, the displayed competence and confidence was due in large part to my previous nursing experience. Credit also goes to my teachers.

During one of the monthly scheduled long distance telephone conversations with my parents and siblings, I familiarized them with the fact that I had successfully delivered babies. Their collective responses made me feel so overly special. I later learnt from my eldest brother that in the home, my name was being used as a mantra, daily reminding them of individual ability and parental expectations. The many friends whom I had made during my training, and who like myself, had migrated to England from different parts of the world, quickly became almost like family. They served as emotional buffers whenever I received a letter or telephone call from my parents, all of which served as an invocation to nostalgia. On so many occasions I had allowed the tears to flow unchecked down my cheeks, when thoughts centered on my sisters and brothers, and wondering what they were doing at that precise moment in time. Were they missing me as much as I was missing them?

With the passage of time, I conscientiously resolved to transform the recurrent bouts of nostalgia into a steely determination to succeed in my studies. Such a plan paid high dividends when six months later, I sat and successfully passed the second part of the Central Midwives Board Examination. I was now a fully qualified midwife, and entitled to use the letters S.C.M (State Certified Midwife) after my name.

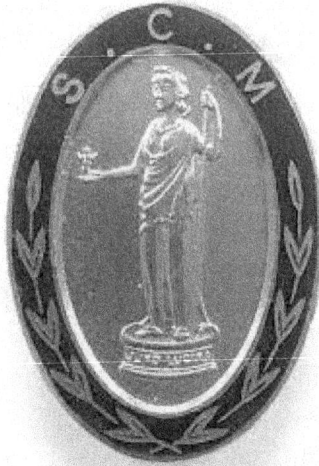

*State Certified Midwife Badge*

Graduation was somewhat bittersweet, as again my parents were unable to travel to London to see me graduate. Concomitantly, to add to my parents' state of joy, my eldest sister had been accepted at a university in the USA to commence studies towards a degree in Business Administration. I sensed a feeling of sadness in my mother's voice as she detailed the good news to me. On inquiring as to the sudden vocal change, she vehemently attributed it to the onset of a likely cold, and jokingly refused to accept the reasons that I proffered as being responsible for the change in her voice.

My growing love for midwifery, and the many radiant faces that surrounded each delivery were not enough to keep me in check, or quell the fire of ambition. I was happy to be trained in an era when midwives knew each patient they cared for and delivered. Despite the value and esteem in which I was held both in the hospital and in the district, I still felt academically unfulfilled. A nagging void persisted, growing daily in intensity, as I firmly clung to the well-known adage: ***"If you want to be considered for the test, then you must be better than the rest"***.

Consequently, eight months later I resigned my position as Staff Midwife, in search of yet another qualification ---- one that would prove to be my final quest.

# PSYCHIATRISTS

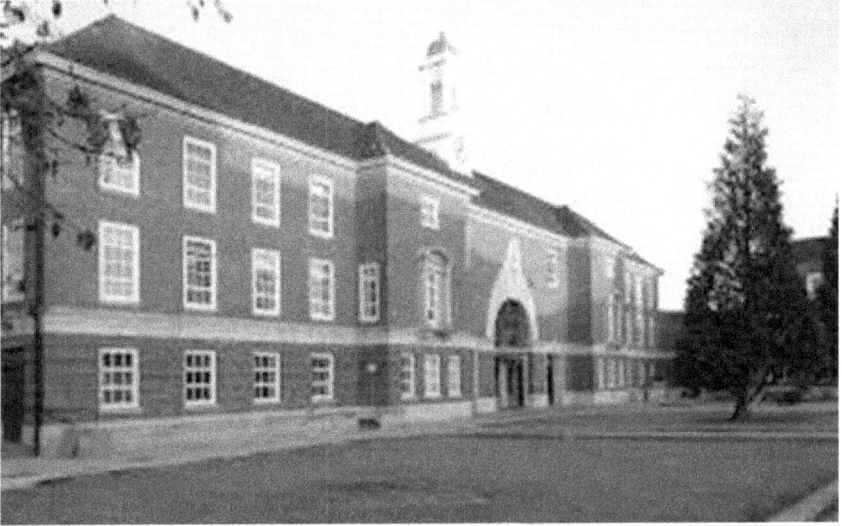

*All Saints Psychiatric Hospital*

It was a bleak winter morning when an iconic London black cab drove me unceremoniously through the iron gates of All Saints Psychiatric Hospital in Birmingham. I would begin my Psychiatric Nurse Training (referred to as Mental Nurse Training), within the confines of this institution, a training of eighteen months duration. The training period had been shortened on account of my prior acquisition of Nursing registration. Slowly the driver brought the cab to a halt in front of a building with the word Main Administration boldly printed above one of its doors, whereupon, he immediately got out and lost no time in opening the door for me to do the same.

I stood nervously on the sidewalk, watching the back of the cab become a speck down the same winding cobblestone driveway which I had travelled a few minutes earlier. Standing uprightly on either side of me, as if keeping guard or waiting for me to make the next move, were my two suitcases. Throwing a furtive glance around my immediate surroundings, and muttering a hastily contrived request under my breath for some form of divine intervention, I slowly approached the closed wooden door that stood before me.

All the buildings on the extensive property presented an eerie appearance, like haunted houses scattered over the vast pristine grounds. My initial impression only further exacerbated my anxiety, especially since I was so consciously aware of the fact that for the next eighteen months, this was going to be the place that I would be calling home. I tried my utmost to compose myself so as not to display the feeling of dread and nervousness that was gradually enveloping me. I felt my knees literally shaking, and the palms of my hands becoming sweaty, as I approached the door of the building. I possessed very little knowledge of psychiatry, except that psychiatric hospitals were places where the insane were locked away for the protection, comfort and security of the public at large, as well as for themselves. Had I unwittingly crossed the thin line between sanity and insanity, and was now in need of a psychiatrist rather than psychiatric training? Had I overextended myself? What should I do? Immediate answers were nowhere to be found.

The door opened before I even had time to knock, revealing a rather robust woman with a somewhat shy look on her face. In a distinctly masculine voice she introduced herself as Miss Todd, the Home Warden. "How odd, Miss Todd", I thought, quickly turning my face aside to conceal a silent grin. After a brief inquiry into my trip to the hospital, to which I gave a laconic explanation, she handed me a set of keys, and a floor plan with my residence and room number circled in black. How ominous!, immediately realizing that my residence was one of the seemingly haunted looking buildings on the hospital grounds. I felt the urge to run away but sadly my feet felt incapable of moving.

Miss Todd inquired as to whether I had any questions or concerns, and upon receiving a negative response, she immediately assured me that my suitcases would be taken to my room. Questions?

I repeated under my breath. She had to be joking. Yes, I had questions, lots of them, but none that she was capable of answering. I am still puzzled as to how after such a brief initial encounter I was able to discern that she was somewhat inept and unfit for such a position-confirmation of which would come during my stay. For the next year and a half, while her life would be unavoidably linked to that of mine, nonetheless, would have little else in common.

Walking to the residence, I carefully perused the floor plan that Mrs. Todd had given me, all the while from time to time, looking over my shoulder for some unknown reason. Slowly, I opened the door to my room, clutching the door knob and delaying my entrance, leaving it partly ajar to allow any unknown or unwelcome presence to make its exit. I was sending a clear message that the new resident had arrived, prepared and ready for immediate occupancy.

The layout of the new living quarters bore an uncanny resemblance to the two that I had occupied during my previous training sessions. I concluded that all hospitals and nurses' living quarters in England were designed according to the same specifications and perhaps by the same architect with a penchant for the dreary.

My thoughts on hospital architecture soon gave way to much-needed sleep. I needed rest so badly that only on awakening the following morning did I realize that I had not eaten since lunch the previous day. I needed sleep more than alimentation. Anyway, here I was, eighteen months less one day to go. My countdown would feature days, weeks, hours, minutes and every second. A folded piece of paper peeping out from under my door suddenly caught my attention, which on opening turned out to be notification of a 9.00 a.m. appointment the following morning to be fitted for nursing uniforms. It was already Thursday, and the Preliminary Training Session (P.T.S) was scheduled to begin on

Monday, therefore it was imperative that this appointment be kept. Not only did I have to be present on the first day of training school, but above all properly uniformed.

In the sewing room I was measured and given my nursing uniforms, a packet of three nursing caps, and six aprons. Taking my carefully wrapped package, which I signed as having received, I furtively looked around wondering if some of the workers in the sewing room were actual psychiatric patients, given their displayed body movements and occasional odd facial grimaces. Leaving the room I saw three of the workers waving their hands at me in an almost clown-like fashion. I nevertheless kept my gaze straight ahead, deciding in my best interest not to respond to the farewell gestures.

The classroom instructor Mr. Richard Bugg, unceasingly drummed it into the craniums of the nursing students, that psychiatry differed in its entirety, from all other nursing disciplines --- a fact that he insisted should always be remembered. Those were the first words uttered to the class of 33 students, after personal self- introduction, and supplying of background details. In a somewhat authoritative voice, he bellowed, "The brain is a strange and moving vehicle, the moistest organ in the body, and once damaged can never be restored to its original form or function." He entreated us to never forget this fact, even if, over time, we forget other things that he will teach us.

Somehow or other, the manner in which Instructor Bugg handled the topic of the brain, its anatomical functions and various mental disorders, aroused in me a slight fear of psychiatry and all that it represented. In a continued effort to be open to whatever was to come, I sought solace by delving into my textbooks at every available opportunity. I wanted to learn everything there was to learn about psychiatry, in a desperate bid to pay homage to Mr. Bugg's inauspicious warnings.

My continued presence as a psychiatric nurse-in-training, brought in its wake the unsettling feeling that I was continually battling an unknown opponent, and one against whom I was a poor match. Nevertheless, I was inwardly determined that fear would not serve as a contributory factor.

One day during my training I was assigned to a Staff Nurse who was responsible for the medication administration on the Unit. As she commenced her dispensatory duties, it was blatantly obvious from her actions, and facial appearance that my presence was not a desired one, thereby making the patients by default the recipients of all her verbal outpourings. As I followed the nurse, I mentally reminded myself as to the reason for being there and above all so far from home. I thought to myself, "I am supposed to be here to learn". So, without any further ado, I cleared my throat and in an inquiring tone said, "Can you tell me why we are giving these tablets to this patient, and what will they do for him?" I can still remember her drawing herself up over her belt, appearing to be almost the size and shape of the Goodyear Blimp and bellowing in a gruff voice: "Nurse, you are not here to ask questions, you are here to do the work, so get on with it." Seemingly, the expected attitude was to do exactly as I was told and not to ask any questions, or at least of a certain type.

Across the hall from my room in the dormitory, I befriended Daisy a student nurse who hailed from Rhodesia, and who was in the final months of her psychiatric training. On discovering that I had already successfully completed both my General Nursing and Midwifery Training, she regarded me as a genius of sorts. We were daily visitors to each other's room once we had finished work, becoming almost inseparable as time progressed. The time spent together was not restricted solely to social chatter, but instead was productively spent, with her studying for her forthcoming finals, while I read my textbooks, and increased my knowledge through listening to her answers from the exercises in the textbook.

As our friendship progressed, Daisy confided in me, outlining from a nursing perspective what could safely be termed a "survival strategy." She was quite adamant when she stated that in order to "fit in" on some wards I should keep my mouth shut particularly if I saw things that I did not like. No speak!" she intoned. "You do not have to join in anything that you do not like, but you must never report any staff". No See! "If you report people you will never be trusted, and even your own nursing colleagues will encourage violent patients to beat you up, and if you are ever in trouble with a violent patient, they will not come to your rescue."

Daisy said that most nurses from General Hospitals oftentimes have trouble fitting in with nurses from other disciplines especially psychiatry. They see things happening on the Unit, disagree, and start reporting fellow staff, sometimes with serious outcomes. They behave as if they are the self- appointed Gestapo of the profession. "Remember, it takes a special kind of someone to work in a mental hospital," she cautioned.

Not only Daisy's words, but the manner in which they were spoken, would remain with me forever. I was convinced that Daisy had my best interest at heart and wanted to see me do well even when she would be no longer around.

Like most other nursing students, I soon realized that not only was I totally ignorant of mental disorders, but I now needed to unlearn all my previously –held concepts and notions about insanity. I was in concurrence with Mr. Bugg that psychiatry was a nursing specialty; in fact, the only specialty that was forcing me to closely and regularly examine myself alongside my fellow humans.

There was so much that I did not understand, and had yet to know about people, and what determined their way of thinking, acting and behaving. There were times when some of the behaviours of my peers and even that of my own, very closely mimicked those who had been diagnosed as being mentally insane. While some patients clinically displayed the reasons justifying why psychiatric help was sought in their cases, or why the public needed to be protected from them, others puzzlingly showed a degree of thinking that was clearly superior to those "sane" folks on the outside. The lines between sanity and insanity were not clearly evident, or at best were ill defined, and I certainly needed assistance in knowing and seeing the difference between the two.

As my studies gradually progressed and I seriously felt, as if on the verge of gaining a better understanding of psychiatry and its various terminologies, an incident would occur leaving me with the impression that I that either witnessed a hallucination, or that I was plain deluded, and in need of redefining the term "mental illness".

During an admission interview, I can vividly recall the conversation between psychiatrist and soon-to-be admitted individual that went thus:

**Psychiatrist:** "Well, Mr. Harrison, what brought you here this time?"

**Patient:** "Doc, I used the tube and the 76A bus from Elms Green. My wife brought me to see you. It was all her idea."

**Psychiatrist:** "Why do you think she brought you?"

**Patient:** "I have no idea, she's always springing surprises on her friends, and you have been a longtime friend of ours."

**Psychiatrist:** "Tell me, how have you been doing lately?"

**Patient:** "What do you mean, Doc?"

**Psychiatrist:** "Just tell me, what have you been up to? Tell me anything!"

**Patient:** "Last week I built a birdhouse with my grandson, visited my mom in Chelmsford, and I am up to Chapter 6 in the book I am reading. Another thing, Doc, I think that the bloke across the road from our house is up to no good. He doesn't work yet has a big car, and is always talking to himself. Don't you think he needs to see you? Shall I tell him?"

No further dialogue occurred between the psychiatrist and the patient. I recall the patient protesting loudly as he was forced to exchange his outdoor garments for the identifiable hospital attire. His wife stood by in deep conversation with the psychiatrist, every now and then. casting the odd glance in her husband's direction

As students Mr. Bugg repeatedly quizzed us on the definitions of illusion, delusion, phobia, and other psychiatric terminologies. I had the definition of a delusion down pat, and from time to time as if on cue, I would blurt out the definition. It did not matter one bit, since I was in a psychiatric environment, where normalcy remained somewhat of an unknown. To this day, and even after prolonged residence in different continents, I can still recall the definitions verbatim ----- a **delusion**: a false belief held fixedly in the face of reason, **illusion**--: a misinterpretation in the absence of an outside stimuli.

As my training progressed, days, turning into weeks and ultimately months, I assiduously developed an interest in carefully reading the admission history, the psychiatric history and observing the patient, in an endeavor to see if I could arrive at the same final diagnosis as that of the admitting psychiatrist.

One evening, shortly after 6.00 p.m., a bearded, somewhat disheveled and handcuffed young man, appearing to be in his mid-twenties, was brought to our Locked Treatment Unit, following his earlier passage through the court system. He was being admitted under the order of Her Majesty's Pleasure, which meant that he would be imprisoned, for an indeterminate period of time until the Queen of England (Parole Board of England acting on her behalf) decided that he no longer posed a risk and was ready to be released. Notice regarding his admission had been transmitted from the Main Admitting Office to the Unit, with no stated reason, except that he had been seen by a judge in court. I looked on as this new admission was ushered into the sitting area, where the transporting police quickly and surreptitiously removed his handcuffs. He was then taken to his room by two male staff, supervised while undressing, then had his personal belongings checked and locked away. Both the police and the accompanying court documents identified him as Harold Bragg, but the patient vehemently denied this as being his name, claiming that he had never heard it before. This response remained unchanged each time the question of identification was raised, and it was becoming increasingly evident that he was desperately trying to control his anger when responding. He repeatedly affirmed, "My name is Jesus or Geesus.

As was the routine admission procedure, the psychiatrist conducted the admission interview. The patient was extremely cooperative throughout the procedure, although appearing somewhat guarded at times. Occasionally, he would cast an upward gaze mumbling in an almost inaudible tone as if communicating with an unseen other being. On being asked if he was seeing or hearing things he denied both visual and auditory hallucinations, reiterating once again, "My name is "Jesus " " or "Geejus ". I found it strange that despite the repeated questioning no one had thus far elicited his surname.

The conducted interviewing session went thus:

**Psychiatrist:** "What is your name?"

**Patient:** "Jesus, but you can call me Geesus."

**Psychiatrist:** "Do you know Harold Bragg?"

**Patient:** "No."

**Psychiatrist:** "Have you ever heard the name Harold Bragg?"

**Patient:** "Yes, since my arrival here I have heard the nurses and some other people over there asking for him from time to time. his name, but I have not met him personally."

**Psychiatrist:** "So, your name is Jesus?"

**Patient:** "Yes, but you can call me Joe for short—Jesus On Earth".

**Psychiatrist:** "Do you know any other person called Jesus?"

**Patient:** "Yes."

**Psychiatrist:** "Tell me, what do you know about him?"

**Patient:** "Well, I don't know a lot about him, except that he lives in some place called Haven. I do not have his exact address."

**Psychiatrist:** Have you ever met him?

**Patient:** No.

**Psychiatrist:** "Thank you very much."

One torrid summer day, a pair of Bobbies (English policemen) were seen struggling to get a fairly middle aged and bespectacled individual out of their police van. From all appearances he appeared to be getting the better of them both. Despite this visible display of non-compliance, there was no retaliatory aggression either in deeds or gestures made by the policemen. Through the window I could see them pleading with him to exit the vehicle, even offering their hands as if to facilitate the exiting process. He began to comply with their request, and soon the trio were headed in the direction of the Emergency Admission Unit. He appeared to be still arguing with the Bobbies, but at least he was following their directives. The individual in question eventually ended up being admitted to my unit. As related by the Bobbies the rationale for his admission was as follows:

Outside a grocery store in the village was a sign clearly displayed for all to see-- "Beat the Heat! Take home a case of Coke today!" Stacked next to the sign were several cases of canned and bottled Coke. The shopkeeper had summoned the police after the individual was seen leaving the store with an unpaid case of Coke. The miscreant had become somewhat belligerent and difficult to reason with when confronted and asked to either return the items or pay for them.

He vehemently maintained that there was no sign indicating cost or demanding payment.

How true! I reasoned. In his seemingly, mentally disorganized state, he was challenging the subliminal messages conveyed by advertising. In a similar manner of reasoning, he pointed out that clearly the sign was inviting the public to take home a case of Coke, and in like manner the price should also be displayed. According to him the advertisement was misleading, and he hated people playing what he angrily referred to as "mind games."

Granted, the word "free" did not appear in the advert, but then again no further details followed the offer to take home a case of Coke. He was only going along with what had been written.

There is a well-known saying, "Blessed are the cracked, for they let in the light." Perhaps our Coke thief was letting in a little "light" so that others might see.

As a novice to the world of psychiatry and uncategorized mental disorders, I racked my brain trying to decide where in the Diagnostic and Statistical Manual of Mental Disorders (D.S.M.) did this type of behavior fall. Was there any sense behind this seeming non sense? Was it an illusion or a delusion? I was uncertain, but I intended to leave the decision and diagnosis to those individuals holding the title of Psychiatrist, and who had studied mental illnesses and its processes for more years than I had or ever would. Psychiatry at its very best would always remain puzzling to me. The statement made by Mr. Bugg at the commencement of my training now resonated.

Readers should not get the impression that psychiatric wards are all barrels of laughter. No, this is not always the case. There are some patients who are pretty much having an awful time of it, where the illness serves as a tormenting agent, as in the case of schizophrenics experiencing auditory hallucinations that more often than not causes the sufferer to carry out self-harmful or even deadly acts.

There is a well-known saying in psychiatric circles, "Blessed are the cracked, for they let in the light." Perhaps our Coke thief was letting in a little "light" so that others might see.

35

Despite the struggle to fully comprehend the seeming intricacies of psychiatry, I fully immersed myself in my studies, worked hard and successfully completed my training. Daisy had left the hospital some time ago, having passed her final examination. She had followed in my footsteps, though in a somewhat reverse order, going on to begin Registered Nurse Training at a hospital situated in the north of England. Despite her departure we still maintained regular communication, and she was overjoyed when I told her that I had passed my final examination. I took the opportunity once again to thank her for those invaluable words of caution that she had imparted to me, and which had served me so well throughout my entire training period.

Following graduation from All Saints Psychiatric Hospital, my last English training school, I began to set my sights on foreign soil. The bug of migration had once again stung me, and for some inexplicable reason Canada became my migratory choice. Although I harbored a slight dislike for working in chaotic, and dangerous situations, I nevertheless thoroughly enjoyed talking and working with the individuals I had encountered and nursed, even in situations that warranted calling a code in order to ensure patient and staff safety, or a return to normalcy. Collectively, they had demonstrated, in the simplest manner, the unpredictable nature of life, and that as humans, any of us suddenly or gradually could lose our hold on reality. In their own individual way each patient under my care, taught me true compassion for other human beings, especially those incapable of helping themselves.

# CHAPTER 4
# UNHOLY TRINITY

> "And in the end, it is not the years in your life that count, It's the life in your years".
>
> — *Abraham Lincoln*

I sought and obtained part-time employment at Daniel Nursing home, situated in Ipswich a seaport town on the outskirts of Suffolk, in eastern England. This 150-bed nursing home, was divided into four one storey units of which Pastime House was included, and at the time was renowned for its cutting-edge technology in geriatrics. I worked in Pastime House along with two other State Enrolled Nurses (Nursing Assistants), three Auxiliary Nurses (Nurses' Aide), a ward cleaner, and a kitchen maid. The labour demands were certainly no pastime. Nothing was quite the same on any given day, given the constraints of looking after a group of people which included many who were confused, immobile, and incontinent (a triad of conditions known in the sector as "the unholy trinity"). On Tuesdays in the mid-afternoon there was a sing –along session hosted by the local branch of Sweet Adeline. Bingo was held every Wednesday evening following clearing away of the supper dishes. Visits to the on-site hairdresser were scheduled for Thursdays. There was always a movie on Friday nights, and patients had once weekly shampoo, shower and hand/ foot care or a combination of both if warranted.

The less mobile and very ill residents consumed their meals in their rooms under the supervision and assistance of the nurse's aides. About a third of the residents were on antidepressant medication, seemingly to help them cope with being there------- a sad irony. Once a year, usually in the summer, a few of the more physically- able residents took a bus outing to the flea market in the adjoining town.

Apart from the scheduled outings and games and movie night, life in the nursing home was monotonous, uneventful and somewhat confined.

Allow me to give you a walking tour.

Follow me into the Day Room where the residents are encouraged to spend their wakeful hours. It may be difficult for you as it was for me, not to be shocked at the way the patients are seated. Most are dozing; some are slumped over in their chairs, others using the trays attached to their wheelchair as head rests or pillows. One extremely fragile and gaunt resident, 95-year-old Elsie Thicke, gives the impression that she is being swallowed up by her armchair, her thin elbows barely poking up over the armrests.

Paulette, the Unit Charge Nurse on duty, is carrying out her rounds of the rooms, where some of the lesser mobile residents are lying in bed watching the television, or in politically correct terms, looking at the screen.

Her approach and interaction with each patient is distinct and effective—playful and argumentative with some of the more alert and lively, tender, compassionate, and kind with the sick. She begins to spoon water into Millie's mouth. "How are you today? Do you still have that frog in your throat? "You need to drink, so please drink now," she pleads, adding approvingly when Millie accepts some orange squash, "Lovely lass." The corridor is noisy with the sound of frequent raspy coughing, and the blended noise of televisions each on a different channel, all at volumes suited for the hearing impaired.

"How are you today?" Paulette inquires at every room. "Not too good, ducky," many of the residents reply. "Very, very poorly." She comforts them, "Don't worry dears," don't worry."

On completing the medication round, Paulette carefully verifies that the trolley is locked and parks it in its reserved place. Next she sits down to do the paperwork. She will return to check discreetly at each resident's door at least three or even more times before finishing her shift.

As she begins her charting Paulette says, "Aging is a natural process, but sometimes it can be a very complicated one."

I was assigned to care for an elderly resident named Betty, who from the nursing report was extremely ill, in the final stage of Hodgkin's lymphoma. Her present condition required that I spend lengthy periods of time at her bedside carrying out special care. I massaged her shoulders and stroked her hair. "Never mind," I whisper gently, while cleaning her mouth with a small pink medical sponge attached to a cotton bud. She is edentulous, and her face has fallen inwards where her mouth used to be. Her eyes remained tightly shut, and the occasional sound, emitting from her partly –closed mouth could be a sigh or a moan. I calmly reassured her that I was there, introducing myself as Nurse Yvonne.

Formerly, the nursing profession meant extreme physical work, with strict adherence to deadlines and time constraints. At regularly – scheduled intervals patients were turned and repositioned in bed to relieve pressure points, certain areas such as the heels, knees, elbows and sacral areas were vigorously massaged and barrier cream applied. Even the pillows were fluffed and turned over so that after the patient would lie in a changed position on a fresh side of the pillow. In this way we were fully aware, among other things, of the patient's skin integrity, and if there was any particular problem that needed to be addressed.

Today, nurses attend university, and are more paper than people oriented. In a healthcare system where profit seems to take precedence over good practice, what has been truly lost are the qualities that matter most to a patient—compassion and hands-on care. Reaffirming the caring nature of nursing, and actively promoting these behaviors may be effective in making the profession a more attractive and appealing career choice.

# CHAPTER 5
# INJUSTICES

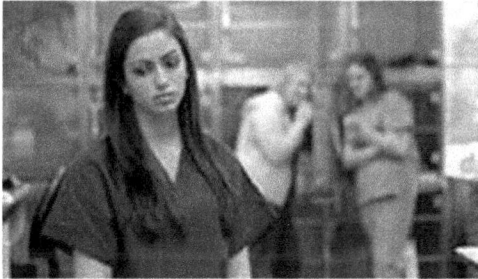

Old state nursing home in New York City was known to hire nurses of a certain caliber, a fact that I learned long after I had accepted employment there. I remember as a new nurse being eager to test all my nursing skills to ensure that any assigned patient received the best care along with my undivided attention. I really thought that I was doing my best, but there were occasions when these displays of my best efforts were met by loud and public outbursts, "Would you cut it out? Stop mollycoddling them! "There are lots of other things to do". There was absolutely no regard for the fact that although a part time employee, I was nevertheless a senior nurse.

Staff were not encouraged to spend too much time at the bedside of any patient, unless it was task-related. The unspoken and accepted protocol was--- simply go to the bedside, carry out the task or procedure and exit on completion. No time for chitchatting or listening to tales of woe. Any patient in real distress, would ring the bell. The real problem was the constant telling off that the novices received from the "experienced" for doing not only what they were taught to do, but what they also thought was a good job.

Do not for a nano second harbour the thought or belief that it is only the young nurses that get eaten by their superiors. Rather, they are the ones that get eaten more often. As one nurse aptly put it, "the young get eaten because they are tender". When a pack mentality takes over, it is common to see and hear two or more nurses munching away on a colleague of similar age or experience. With the passage of time, improved experience and professional maturity, it became apparent that not only did nurses eat their young, but they were certainly not selective of what they ate.

Nursing instructors also form part of the "eating system." albeit with a differentiating tool. They have been known to berate students for not coming to classes, despite being ill and providing a doctor's note. Another nursing student reported missing her stage because she had gone to the Emergency Department with suspected cholecystitis (inflammation of the gallbladder). The next day, in front of all the other nurses, she was told, "You had better get your priorities in order."

When teaching new nurses, preceptors often exclaim, "See one, do one, teach one" while demonstrating a new procedure, anything from sterile "gloving" to the hanging of blood for transfusion. They will demand that the new nurse observe them carrying out the procedure technique, perform unassisted, and then show it to someone else. Preceptors have been known to make disparaging comments to the new nurse when she fails to carry out the procedure correctly. The student nurse would also become the main item during the preceptor's break periods, as she ensures that her colleagues are all aware of the student nurse's shortcomings.

One day, the unit was extremely busy due to having more admissions in a shorter time than usual. The Nurse in Charge requested that my colleague take the next admission as I was otherwise occupied. Without a moment's hesitation and within earshot of the Charge Nurse, my colleague looked me directly in the face and said, "If you cannot handle the workload, then change floors". I was completely surprised and rendered speechless by such behavior, moreover from my peers. I walked away from the desk and hurriedly made my way to the bathroom, my usual refuge when my lacrimal sacs became activated. Oh!, how I wish that I was not so young, not so tender, but hard enough to give her immediate gastric upset, and bring about a forced menu change.

Once, while working on the medical floor, I overheard Nurse Bitchin telling my colleague Faith, who had joined our team one week earlier, "I did all your work, I should get your paycheck." I felt horrible for her. It was so reminiscent of behaviors that I had been subjected to previously. Faith later confessed to me that she had asked Nurse Bitchin many questions, mainly to ensure that she was carrying out the tasks correctly. However, she had fully completed her assignments unassisted. It was obvious even to the visually myopic that nurses nurture patients, but never each other. Some veteran nurses are of the belief that such an approach is a satisfactory means of "toughening up" the novices. Abuse and insult only decreases confidence and competence. Conversely, doctors, paramedics, physiotherapists and other members of the healthcare team do not display insensitive behaviour towards the nurses

It was the end of my shift, and I listened as Destiny, one of my co-workers, was being hassled over the phone for the second time that day.

For some strange or diabolical reason the Staff Nurse just seemed to have it in for her, with no evident letup in sight. Poor Destiny was not only the main course, but the dessert as well. "Why have you not done this?" "Why have you not done that?" "Have you given the drug?" "Started the I.V? Got the lab results? Called the dietician? Notified the resident?" For valid reasons, Destiny was not able to complete some of these tasks. She was prepared under calmer and less dictatorial conditions to give the Staff Nurse a detailed report of the completed and incomplete tasks along with her explanations. This nurse was known to boast about giving the interns—the doctors in training— the new nurses- the old nurses all a hard time and apparently enjoyed doing so. No one had ever knowingly made any attempt to challenge her at her game, or even forced her to change her strategy. Everyone pussyfooted around her, trying their level best to remain on her good side.

Angel, the night nurse on our Medical Surgical Unit, had just undergone an extremely hectic shift. At 5 a.m., a recently- admitted sixty-year-old female patient suddenly started to go sour, responding poorly to rigorous nursing interventions. As the senior nurse, in addition to being the assigned nurse, Angel had spent the greater part of her shift carrying out the expected procedures: carefully recording the vital signs, frequently turning and positioning, monitoring every response to administered treatment, and notifying the doctor as necessary.

The carrying out of these nursing duties rendered her somewhat incapable of fully caring for some of the other patients entrusted to her care. During the handing over of the night report to the oncoming shift, one of the nurses who had just arrived on duty, angrily inquired as to the reason why a patient under Angel's care had not been shaved for surgery. The question was blatantly redundant, almost unworthy of a response. The oncoming Nurse in Charge was fully aware of the demanding night that Angel had experienced, and in an openly sincere manner, had accepted the proffered reasons for the non-completion of some assigned nursing duties.

Nursing is an extremely difficult and demanding profession, as we are required to work odd shifts, public holidays, and exceedingly long hours. Inherent in each shift is the element of unpredictably and ordered chaos. In a second, a formerly stable patient could become unstable oftentimes with fatal results. The phones would ring non-stop, doctors, residents and even medical students would appear unexpectedly on the unit, or fail to when they have been called and are most needed. The timing of off-unit tests and procedures are coordinated with scheduled nursing activities. To further compound this potential maelstrom, the absence of a staff member requires that the remaining nurses pick up the slack by having extra patients added to their workload, instead of finding a replacement. Nursing can safely be likened to a never -ending roller coaster ride.

Similar episodes of such behaviours and attitudes have been recounted by my nursing colleagues employed in other hospitals, and to which I can attest having been the victim of lateral hostility at the hands of my peers. New nurses have repeatedly and continually spoken of the treatment they have received from senior nurses, who have blatantly refused to render assistance when asked, and have loudly corrected the junior nurse oftentimes in the presence of patients and visitors. These public displays of belittlement have often left the unsuspecting onlooker with the impression that it was done to show where and with whom the superior knowledge lay.

This harsh and sometimes abusive treatment of new nurses was previously the dirty secret of nursing, but time has gradually forced it out into the open. Now more than ever, it is imperative that this problem be publicly acknowledged and discussed, as it is sometimes difficult for nurses to accept and admit that their actions and attitudes could be hurting each other.

During nursing school, one of the nursing instructors postulated that nursing is seen by the public as an honest, credible, and trusted profession. The term "nurse" then becomes an oxymoron. While nurses are placed on a pedestal for being compassionate, caring, and supportive, at the same time they are the perpetrators of negative approaches, indifferent treatment and hostility to their very own.

In Canada, I had the good fortune to work for an employment agency on an as-needed basis. This permitted me to work on various nursing units in several hospitals, which from time to time afforded me the pleasurable experience of joining a team on units that were well managed, effective and efficient. There were also other Units that lacked communicative leadership, collaborative team spirit and basic professionalism. Ironically and unsurprisingly, I am yet to hear or witness a nurse speaking up when a fellow nurse is humiliated, but on the other hand will advocate and speak up for a patient without hesitation. This contradiction is puzzling.

While carrying out a practicum as a student nurse at Berry General Hospital, on entering the room I espied a middle-aged Asian woman sobbing loudly and uncontrollably. She was sitting on the edge of the bed, slightly hunched over, with her lips quivering as she tried to speak in response to my questioning. I reassuringly placed my hands on her shoulders and waited patiently as she made an evident effort to compose herself. "Please tell me what is the matter?" I again implored.

Awaiting her response, I assumed that she may have been suffering from intractable back spasms, a reopening wound, or perhaps severe abdominal pain. The loud sobbing slowly decreased in volume morphing into a spasmodic sniffling, and, turning to me with reddened eyes and tear-moistened cheeks, Kleenex in her hands poised for action, she whispered almost in an inaudible tone, "That nurse was so mean and downright nasty to me." Pausing for a while, looking slowly around, and then almost as if gaining vocal strength from an invisible source, she loudly blurted out "What's wrong with her, I did her nothing?" Apparently this patient was not in pain, but was instead crumbling from caustic words and harsh treatment, meted out by a nurse.

For a lingering moment I mentally empathized with her, thinking to myself, if only she knew that she was not the only victim of such rough treatment.

It had been a quiet evening on the gynecological ward, despite being extremely hectic at the start of the shift., but later calmed down as the evening progressed. The patient in Bed 9 had been admitted following the termination of a 14-week pregnancy. Her call bell was activated and through the intercom I could hear her tearfully requesting a painkiller. Her words were muffled but a plea of desperation for help was evident, given the tone of her voice. Almost fifteen minutes or more elapsed, and once again her call bell was activated. Although I was not assigned to this patient, I immediately responded, and went directly to her room to further investigate. She was curled up in bed in an almost fetal-like position, writhing in evident agony, complaining of severe pain, transient nausea and requesting that something be given quickly for the intractable pain she was experiencing. As I left the room, I reassured her that I would immediately bring the matter to the attention of her assigned nurse, as well as the Charge Nurse, and ensure that she was seen and treatment administered.

On returning to the Nursing Station, I immediately informed the Charge Nurse of the patient's request, painstakingly detailing the condition in which I had found her. With a straight face and in a manner that I will not easily forget for a long time to come, the Charge Nurse responded, "She can wait; if you can kill a child, then you can suffer a bit."

There are, of course, instances when a nurse's kindness and willingness to break rules on behalf of a patient are revealed. In the Psycho-Geriatric Unit, a male patient suffering from dementia and who was occasionally restrained in bed, decided not to remain in his room. The nurses had spent a great part of the evening shift redirecting him from the wrong bed and wrong room and into his bed, all before the incumbents became aware of his unsolicited presence and unwarranted visit.

While sitting in the nursing station, I noticed that Mr. Foole had once again left his bed and had sought refuge in the bed of Miss Howlett. I immediately brought this slightly funny situation to the attention of the senior nurse. As I readied myself to head in the direction of the scene of the infraction, and assist in returning Mr. Foole to his assigned place of rest, I felt a sharp tug on my right arm, forcing me to immediately stop in mid stride. The voice at the end of my arm inquired as to my destination. For a moment I was unable to speak as only a few minutes earlier in the best Queen's English I had familiarized her with the illicit behavior of Mr. Foole and Miss Howlett. What did she fail to understand? Then with a half grin, and a slight wink, she asked, "Do you have a boyfriend?" Interpreting my silence as an affirmative response, she thereupon entreated me to leave Mr. Foole alone, as he also needed a friend.

Stunned not only by this response but also by the visible absence of any meaningfully significant intervention on her part, I thereupon changed direction and walked slowly towards the Nursing Station, refusing to dwell on the possibly unfolding amorous situation and emanating reactions. I felt that in the interest of team unity, not to mention personal reputation, my lips would remain forever sealed where this issue was concerned, an action that would lessen, or even eradicate my likely vulnerability to being eaten. And it was possible that the supervising nurse had shown wisdom I did not appreciate at the time. Additionally, should any form of interaction or intimacy take place between these two senior citizens, Providence thankfully would be on their side. At their age, conception would not only be unthinkable but also equally impossible.

There are occasions when the way nurses communicate with patients can create a sense of devaluation on the part of the patient. Nurses have been overheard disparaging patients by using baby talk. As one patient related, "The nurse talked to me like I was a child, which not only belittled me but also gave the impression of insincerity." Another patient related his analogous interaction, "This nurse made ironic remarks about an experience". I was told to choose a number between one and ten and to give her an answer regarding my level of pain. When I gave her the number and told her how much pain I was in, she immediately bellowed, "Surely you cannot be in that much pain, for if you were, you'd be in a cold sweat and not as relaxed as you are". Now, you just think about it one more time". This directive heralded the end of her dialogue and intervention.

Patients have complained that nurses themselves have made the decisions regarding their care, totally rejecting their respective input. One patient recounted, "She (the nurse) took control of everything". "When I said we should do like this instead", the nurse said, "You don't understand this". "What are you making a fuss for?' She thought I was trying to correct her, and she was certainly having none of that."

Another patient ruefully lamented, "A nurse neglected to make notes in my chart. She did not write down the information that I told her, which I thought was very important and particularly asked that it be written in my record for my doctor to read". "I think that omitting information is professional negligence, especially when so many people are involved in my care. What is written down is important, as so many things can go wrong with the wrong and missing information, and this really scares me". The patient further added that he had read the medical summary of his nursing care plan, "I saw that they had just copied the old one. It would have been good, if I had been allowed to take part in the planning and evaluation of my care."

Every nurse has a choice either to promote the negative minority or join the positive majority. The time is ever-present to recognize the quiet heroes in our profession -- those who unceasingly do the right thing day after day, investing in the next generation of nurses. It is good to promote what is right about nursing. Instead of eating the young, let us instruct and appreciate them. This would leave the perpetrators no choice but to starve, change their diets, or face severe abdominal discomfort.

Here is another impediment to the profession that I have often heard when receiving reports of patients: "This patient is a "VIP! Suite 34 is a Princess! Room 4309 is Special!"

There is an unspoken requirement that patients who are "special" receive special care and attention, that things be explained more thoroughly and responses to their requests be carried out quickly and efficiently. Management makes more frequent rounds to ensure the V.I.Ps (Very Important Persons) and VSPs (Very Special Persons), receive the very best care. With increasing pressure to improve patient satisfaction scores and with the possible fear of litigation, the most experienced nurses are assigned to the VIPs and VSPs.

Significant attention is given to ensure that the needs of the affluent are satisfactorily met, and during their hospital sojourn only certain nurses become involved in the planning and implementation of their overall nursing care. Meanwhile, in the same unit but in another room is an older male patient, of low socio-economic status, and who resides in a government subsidized housing project. His wife cries openly as she tries to figure out all that is taking place around her, for she wants the best and only the very best for her husband. Due to a lack of understanding of the treatment plan, and a guarded prognosis, she is experiencing some difficulty as to what questions she should ask the team upon her husband's discharge. The medical team is sending the patient home with daily follow-up appointments by the Community Nurse. There is no daily rounding by either management or the medical team, nor is there prior family involvement in his plan of care.

I am often left wondering, at the disparity in patient education and customer service. Why should a patient's "connections" or his social status impact the quality of care received? How can the provision of special care for select individuals be ethically justified? The healthcare system too often fails to advocate for the needs of the indigent while nurses jump to meet the demands of the affluent. Nurses must enter into the fight to eliminate this blatant social injustice and provide the highest quality patient-centered care to everyone we encounter. It is a difficult and often ignored commitment, for many nurses experience a sense of being special when they have been assigned to care for a V.I.P (Very Important Person) or a V.S.P (Very Special Person). Accepting the favoring of the somebodies over the nobodies, the nurse becomes a "curse" and is in the profession only for the purse. She has failed to carry out the true mission for which she has been prepared.

# CHAPTER 6
# NURSE BULLY

> "....reach back and give other folks the same chances that helped you."
> — *Michelle Obama*

Horizontal hostility is defined as hostile, aggressive, and harmful behavior by a nurse or group of nurses toward a co-worker, or group of nurses via attitudes, words and/ or actions. It is also characterized by the presence of a series of undermining incidents over time as opposed to one isolated conflict in the workplace.

Horizontal behavior occurs most frequently among peers ultimately creating a negative work environment, impairing teamwork and compromising patient care, and is often unrecognized and underreported. Nevertheless, it has special implications for students and new graduates who have many questions and require professional development to reach their full potential,

Horizontal behavior can be overt or covert and both are extremely hurtful. Raised eyebrows, sarcastic remarks, or eye rolling can all have a profound effect on teamwork, safety, satisfaction, and staff retention since they are the source of conflict. Sad to say, but in the culture of nursing these behaviors are acceptable, because I believe some nurses lack the skills necessary for effective and constructive peer confrontation.

Today, in many healthcare facilities, administrative hierarchies promote and perpetuate oppressive conditions, such as infrequent uninterrupted breaks or meals, inadequate staffing ratios, limited supplies, and little or no recognition of nurses' ability to think critically. These conditions in their own way all serve as contributory factors to the promotion of horizontal violence.

Charting towards the end of my shift, I could not help but overhear one of my co-workers being hassled over the phone. "Second time today", I thought. "Oh my goodness," Apparently the computer would not release results of tests that had been conducted on a patient, and a nurse in another department was laying all the blame on my colleague. The derogatory remarks were flowing fast and furious like rush hour traffic. I have witnessed similar situations, and experienced hostile treatment myself. In my first nursing job, some of the more senior nurses on the floor told mistruths about the work that I had done, even refusing to assist me at times when I really needed it, and made it their duty to loudly correct my mistakes, especially if there was an audience. When I finally left that work environment, I felt as if I had a large bull's-eye on my back, an open target.

Some researchers opine that because nursing "has its fundamental roots in caring," it is often hard for nurses to admit that they could be hurting one another. However, further studies have shown that most leave their first position within six months, because of some form of verbal abuse or harsh treatment from a colleague.

*Dear Nurse Bully,*

*Why am I putting my feelings into words? Well, I have stored them up for far too long. When I first met you on the unit, I was not yet a nurse, just a second year student. I was almost there. I really thought that you were as nice as you appeared. Now, I know for certain that you were merely putting on a show, especially when the Charge Nurse was in our midst. You repeatedly told me to quit, that I would never make it as a nurse. Every verbal encounter was inundated with disparaging remarks. I really thought that all this was normal.*

*When I learnt that I would be spending six weeks under your tutelage, my entire cardiac and respiratory system decided to behave erratically. I got firsthand experience with apnea, bradycardia, dyspnea, and at times missed heart beats. Instead of teaching me the finer points of nursing, you complained about me behind my back to everyone, even those who did not know of or about me. You wrote me up. You shut me out. You ignored any request I made for help.*

*For several years, Nurse Bully, I retired into my own space. I struggled. I lied a few times because I feared ridicule for not knowing everything. Thank God I didn't make any lethal mistakes. I thought this was normal, but the internal confusion was so great. Our paths crossed a few more times. Sadly, each time I felt as if I was drowning in a pool of confusion, hurt, and frustration. I almost gave up my career completely because I thought this was normal and wanted no part of it. On one occasion, in sheer desperation, I even tried to join you, for I thought that if other successful nurses were tough like that, then I should be, too. I didn't like it. It didn't feel normal at all. I wasn't being myself.*

*I often wonder, Nurse Bully, if you would recognize yourself if I called you out. I doubt it. I believe bullying is solely in the eye of the receiver. Maybe my actions were once perceived as bullying. I do not know. But what I do know is that I don't want this to be accepted as normal anymore. I don't think anyone does, at least not some of my peers that I have spoken with. So please, Nurse Bully, stop and think of what you are saying to your coworkers. Are you helping him or her with your words? Is it necessary to belittle someone just because you feel stressed? Is it too much to give a little guidance now and again? Shouldn't that be our norm?*

*Signed: Nurse Hurt*

There is an epidemic of incivility polluting our healthcare institutions. Here are nurses' personal experiences with incivility.

*"My first nursing job was in a toxic environment. I was warned about the strong personalities there and that I would need to stand my ground to succeed. The worst offenders were two experienced middle-aged nurses who called themselves **"silverheads"**. They both felt it was their responsibility to weed out the new young nurses with disrespect and harassment." They worked similar to a tag team in a wrestling match".*

*"I was a new graduate nurse on a busy Medical-Surgical unit. My preceptor repeatedly criticized me in front of my peers, and once I even overheard two nurses saying they didn't think I would make it another week on the unit. At no time did any of the other nurses offer any help, and I strongly suspected that they were intimidated by my preceptor and did not want to risk getting on her bad side. I was basically alone and adrift in my own sea of confusion and mounting uncertainty. Time may be my saving factor".*

*"The last thing I wanted to do was to make waves during my first week of **"clinicals"**. So there I was, in the nurse's lounge of the oncology unit, trying to 'play or act like a nurse' with my preceptor Lee. I was painstakingly looking at the patient's file and literally trying to figure out what "MAR" meant (let alone its entire contents), when this mean-looking nurse came in and scolded me, or, to be more blunt, tore into me with a vengeance. "You are not supposed to be in here doing work—this area is for relaxing only", she bellowed. Confused, I threw a sheepish glance in the direction of my preceptor, who was now making a thorough examination of the ceiling, as if she had suddenly developed an interest in the intricacies of masonry. This mean nurse continued her tirade of disparaging remarks: "Furthermore, the student nurse shouldn't be taking seats away from actual nurses doing work". I was a bit miffed that my preceptor did not utter a single word to Mildred, one of the nurses present, since she was the one who had initially given me the permission to sit in the room. Completely resolved to avoid any further confrontation, I began to gather my effects and hastily left the room".*

*"Every day after lunch, it was the custom for the nursing students to have a brief mini post-conference with the instructor to discuss any special morning issues before heading back to their respective units. One senior nurse, apparently thought that we had snuck off to Starbucks or something, so I guess she thought she was putting us on blast or getting us in trouble when she exclaimed quite grandiosely (in front of our instructor), "Oh my god! You missed it!! You missed the patient escalating and turning sour! Where have you guys been all this time"?*

*At this point I was pretty much dumbfounded at her behavior, as for the past month or so she had not even afforded us a second glance. My mouth just hung as I gazed upon her as if she had just been certified untreatably insane. She had this self-serving smirk on her face, as if she had really stuck it to us. Imagine the amount of apologies and damage control required on her part when she was informed that we had been with our clinical instructor.*

*"In my first year as a nurse, I began to realize that most of the senior nurses were extremely happy to keep information to themselves, preferring to see a new Registered Nurse fall flat on his or her face, rather than provide or proffer the information to prevent such an occurrence".*

# CHAPTER 7
# HIGH TECH

> "Man is still the most extraordinary computer of all."
>
> — *John Fitzgerald Kennedy*

T he documentation of patient care is a fundamental and critical skill used by nurses to communicate the patient's individual needs and responses to care. Today, information technology (IT) is revolutionizing the healthcare industry and electronic charting is currently the new wave. With this rapid increase in mobile communication access, it is important for nurses to add electronic communication skills to their repertoire of acquired, to- be-acquired, or desirable skills.

Having seen and experienced the distinct advantages of electronic charting over paper charting, I realize there are also some accompanying disadvantages. While a computer makes it extremely easy to keep a chart readable and accessible, it is also equally easy to become accustomed to the ease of a computer. Most computers eventually crash, but healthcare doesn't stop, and nurses must know how to keep going. Not to dash when there's a crash, nor to get themselves in a tizzy and become dizzy. There will simply be a return to hand charting until system restoration is put into effect.

Concern still exists that increasing reliance on information technology will weaken the human connection that is the cornerstone of patient care.

Despite all the evidence of the efficacy of electronic communication, the medical community, particularly at the physician level, has displayed slight reluctance to replace paper records with electronic records. Once again, doctors and nurses are not on the same page.

Due to the freeing of nurses from manual record keeping and other time-consuming chores, information technology has increased nurse-patient interaction, improved the quality of care, and increased patient safety. However, being from the old school, I still fixedly hold the firm belief that face-to-face interactions are still the best way to ensure accurate communication between nurse and client. Are we still really communicating with electronic record keeping? Or is it too easy to get in and out?

Earlier pages in this book have already put to rest the "pecking order" theory and taken bromide as a shield against the recurrent statement and pervasive attitude that "nurses eat their young". Now relief is being sought from the distended abdomen, intractable nausea and vomiting that accompanies consumption of the "young".

The Maternal and Child Care Unit at Mary the Saint Hospital was the first to be selected in the world of advanced technology-- computerization. Once this announcement circulated through the Unit, I began to experience paroxysmal bouts of apprehension, but was solaced by the fact that unlike so many of my peers, I was not approaching keyboard or mouse as a rookie, thanks to my previous exposure to the world of computers, limited though it may have been.

As technological advances multiply exponentially, and new technology and gadgets appear on Nursing Units, there is a new segment of the nursing population that is beginning to experience a behaviour pattern that was previously reserved for new nurses. Reference is being made here to the older seasoned but technologically-challenged veteran nurses. They need the assistance of the young to help them cross or transition to the great electronic divide. One may call this "subtle payback", or "just desserts"

I have not personally witnessed this phenomenon, but I have been on multiple occasions privy to displays of mounting impatience directed this time towards the older nurses. Following the introduction of computers on the Unit, and the advent of electronic charting, some of the younger nurses were requested to assist the lesser capable users. Such a situation gave rise to succinct disdain, especially if the two nurses were not previously enjoying an amicable relationship.

Mayree Jayne overheard one of the nursing veterans loudly calling out from the Charting Room, Double Kick! Double Kick! How do I double Kick! This plea of inquiry was not directed to anyone in particular, but was uttered loud enough to be heard by those within close earshot, and capable of giving a response.

Two young nurses in clear view was making no visible attempt to answer the call for help in changing "double kick" to "double click". It was later related, that one of the young nurses was overheard saying, "Let her ask the mouse, he knows." Maryee Jane confessed that on hearing the desperate cry for help to rectify the kicking or clicking problem, she could picture the look on the faces of the younger nurses, rolling their eyes and smiling inwardly. The younger nurses do not easily forget that some of the older nurses never nurtured nor assisted them when they were newcomers to the floor and also the world of nursing. The first cut is the deepest, and some wounds do take a long time to heal, especially if the perpetrators are still around and on the scene. As nurses we strive collectively in the direction of a tradeoff. The young nurses failed to understand that the veteran nurses were trained and educated long before the advent of the computers, they were basically **"technology immigrants"** facing the onslaught of **"technology citizens"**.

K.T was an older nurse who had been absent from hospital nursing for a few years following the tragic loss of her only son in an automobile accident. She had recently accepted a full-time night duty position, but had to complete an orientation period consisting of four weeks of day duty. K.T had left the unit long before the advent of computer and computer charting. The nurse scheduled to orient K.T was much younger than her, and raised in the electronic tsunami.

Surprisingly, K.T reported that the young nurse was somewhat condescendingly unfriendly towards her. The practice of nurses eating their young or their old is no longer professionally viable or feasible. Older nurses must be embraced, by their fellow nurses, and assisted in removing their fear of technology, which is the face of the future.

Nurses who stand together, will remain a force like no other.

# CHAPTER 8
# ANGELS WITH WHISTLES

"Not all whistleblowers are out of range. Some just merely want to effect change."

— *Anonymous*

When it comes to patient care and ethical actions, most nurses can be trusted, and are exemplars par excellence. While taking responsibility or owning up for one's actions is expected, it is not always easy or considered "acceptable" to report a less professionally responsible colleague.

A Code of Silence exists in the medical profession. While there is wide agreement in the medical community that doctors have an ethical duty to disclose their own errors to patients, there has been less discussion about what physicians should do when they discover that someone else's mistake is that of their colleague. Patients do not always know when their doctor has made a medical error. But other doctors do.

Medicine is not an exact science, and it is changing constantly. Therefore, doctors are not automatically responsible for a wrong diagnosis or an unsuccessful operation, as long as they followed widely-accepted medical practices.

https://educaloi.qc.ca/en/capsules/the-responsibility-of-doctors-for-mistakes/

Most doctors will not tattle on each other even if a wrongdoing has been blatantly committed. However, the culture of the nursing environment encourages nurses to snitch, sell out each other, backbite and sabotage their co-workers. Instead of dealing directly with each other regarding any incident, nurses write up Incident Reports and have Administration handle the matter directly.

A nurse, who worked with me at a local hospital, but in a different department and on a different shift., told me that a certain nurse had been known to set other nurses up. One night she concealed the unit's only oxygen saturation machine **(oximeter)** in an alternative location, so that the nurses who were required to use it would have to inquire as to its whereabouts. Failure to inquire, or to request the machine, was certainly an indication that the patient's oxygen saturation level was not being taken, and she would further check the patient's chart specifically to see if charting had taken place.

I worked on the Postpartum Unit, where on multiple occasions medications would be signed as having been administered to a patient at a certain time, only to have the same patient request a repeat outside of the scheduled delay period. In one instance, the patient was quite adamant that not only had she not received the signed drug, but also not at the time that was stated in the medication book. Instead of confronting the errant individual, and pointing out the unethical aspect of her behavior, other nurses copied the discrepant medication sheets and handed over the copies to management for perusal, investigation and possible disciplinary action.

A mailbox conspicuously situated outside the Head Nurse's door served as a depository for incoming mail, but from time to time tattling peers would surreptitiously slide incident reports under the door, when she was off duty. In this way no one would be able to point an accusatory finger at the transmitter, as the evidence was not visible. One morning on entering her office, the Head Nurse sustained a fractured arm having slid over a mound of envelopes that had been pushed under her door, and which she had failed to notice on entry.

As the Nurse in Charge, it was brought to my attention by a family member that the nurse assigned to their mother never came into the room to carry out any nursing care, or inquire into her state of health. In unison, the husband and daughter loudly announced that they were going to "talk to the doctor about it." Such a move was quite in order, but the Nurse in Charge should also be made aware of their concern. (Doctors have no decision –making authority over nurses; instead they will just refer all such matters to the Head Nurse). I approached the Head Nurse, informing her that the patient's family had requested a meeting. Thankfully, on being made aware of the request she did not solicit any further details from me, as I had resolved beforehand that I desired no part whatsoever in this unfolding situation. Nevertheless, despite the fact that I was only the notifier of the family's request, yet I was accused by the nurse in question of being vindictive, spiteful and wanting to get her fired. None of these accusations bore any semblance to the truth. Neither the nurse in question nor her colleagues ever asked for my version of the incident, which I did not offer anyway. I guess it did not matter. Any nurse, who dares to speak out against a seeming wrong perpetrated by a colleague/working peer, automatically runs the risk of being ostracized and alienated, especially if the Administration has been brought into the picture.

People are not always honest, especially in situations where their livelihood is being threatened. Nursing records and documentation of care have been known to be altered to protect the guilty party, or cover up the wrong done especially when nurses of different ethnicities are involved. Failure to and disclosure of evidence could immediately transform the working environment into a battle zone with **"fighters"** and **"sympathizers"** on the ready.

Nursing codes of ethics bind us to the role of patient advocate thereby compelling us to act when either the rights or safety of a patient is jeopardized. There are personal and professional risks involved in blowing the whistle, but it is necessary today, in a healthcare environment weighed down with fraud, incompetent practitioners and patient safety issues.

In nursing **"whistleblowing"** is a serious action that should be engaged in only after all possible sources and resources have been exhausted, and thoughtful consideration given to the personal and professional ramifications that may ultimately ensue. In essence, a nurse must not engage in an act of whistleblowing hastily or without careful thought and supporting documentation.

Nurses who dare to report problems perpetrated by their peers, regardless of their inherent nature or severity, will undoubtedly find themselves alienated from their colleagues, given the silent treatment, denied certain privileges, and facing various forms of retaliation. Blowing the whistle on abuses in the nursing workplace can be hazardous to employment, and sense of well-being. Fear of retaliation and the stigma associated with being a "troublemaker" or a "whistleblower" are realities that contribute to the underreporting of problems in the healthcare system. It is true that doing the right thing is not always the best thing. But creating and enforcing a culture of silence is detrimental to everyone.

Nursing has been looked upon as one of the most sensitive of professions, consequently, all nursing actions are expected to reflect ethical and moral principles. Dishonesty, especially among qualified nurses, is a legitimate source of concern, as it may spread to other nurses. It is imperative that nurses display morality and character of the highest level, and should be seen on and off the job as prototypes for integrity.

Currently nurses have not been educationally prepared for the ethical distress caused by hostile work environments or the personal and professional risks involved in whistleblowing when discussing patient advocacy, nurse autonomy, or the Code of Ethics for Nurses. Nursing educators need to be proactive and initiate the adoption of a curriculum that includes information on the predictable reprisals that will occur if nurses choose to blow the whistle on misconduct. Nurses, including new graduates and seasoned experts, need to know the risks of reporting wrongdoing in the practice setting and be encouraged to speak up and reminded of the ethical codes of conduct that bind them to safeguard patients from harm

One of the greatest philosophers, Eeyore the donkey of Winnie the Pooh's fame published a book of wise sayings, one of which was: "No matter how good your friends are, and no matter how right you are, they may not stand behind you in a work-related confrontation, and you have to forgive them for that." This is a one-sentence lesson in corporate culture! Eeyore adds two more: "Being right doesn't mean you'll win," and "Blowing the whistle always is painful." He is both right and wise, but sadly Eeyore fails to tell us what to do when it happens.

Early in my nursing career, while employed at All Angels Hospital, I secretly admired a nurse with whom I was privileged to work alongside, and my admiration daily increased as I watched her going about her nursing tasks. Without any doubt she was the favorite of the floor, always managing to get her work done way ahead of her other colleagues. The doctors also praised her, repeatedly remarking about her nursing capabilities, enthusiasm, and cheerful countenance. The nursing notes and charting of the other nurses paled in comparison to hers. Clearly, she was the exemplar as other nurses experienced difficulty from time to time in completing their assignments in a timely manner.

Suddenly, and quite unexpectedly, the truth behind her capable and efficient nursing veneer came to light, thereby ruining her reputation. She had painstakingly documented giving a patient a complete bed bath, assisting with oral hygiene, and even supervising the patient in carrying out respiratory exercises. However, the patient was later overheard asking when would she be washed. She became furious on being told that, according to the written documentation of her assigned nurse, she had already received a wash. Becoming plainly angrier and in defense of her mental cognition, she stated her resentment of the staff treating her as if she was either crazy or suffering from Alzheimer's. It was charted that the procedure had been carried out earlier in the shift, even to the point of stating that the patient had fully enjoyed the wash.

It was also revealed in the case of another patient that the same nurse had charted on the urinary output of the patient, several days after the indwelling catheter had been removed. To worsen such an already deceptive situation, she had even brazenly charted about the volume, odor, and colour of the patient's urine. No longer was it a mystery why she was able to complete her assignment well in advance of her peers. The truth was revealed at its root.

There are nurses who claim to have flushed intravenous infusions, when there were none to be flushed, or charted vital signs that followed the exact data pattern as those of previous nurses, despite obvious clinical changes in the patient's condition. On several occasions, more than I care to recall, I have witnessed mentally competent patients attest that their assigned nurse(s) had not carried out the assessments as noted in their charts. Sadly, there are times when a patient complaint is ignored. Moreover, a complaint is pursued, depending on the nurse involved and the position she occupies within the peer acceptance group on the unit.

The lingering question is whether nurses eventually absorb the "body of knowledge" and become honest over a period of time, or whether some degree of future research should be seriously devoted to finding an answer or a solution. It would be cynical at best to believe that all nurses are somewhat deceptive, for there are those who honestly live up to the demands and expectations of the profession.

One particularly hectic evening on a unit with which I was totally unfamiliar, the nurse went off duty, leaving me with only a tape-recorded end-of-shift report, and seven patients with whom I was also completely unfamiliar. I immediately telephoned the Nursing Supervisor explaining my situation to her, in the hope of receiving some form of advice, support or intervention. She voiced support for my expressed concerns, but claimed that she was unable to do anything, as her hands were tied. She failed to elaborate on how or why her hands were tied. I then asked if this matter should be brought to the attention of the hospital administration. Without hesitation, she told me in an unpleasant voice, "There will be no meeting, and if you want to keep your job, you will keep your mouth shut and not raise such concerns again."

In some cases, especially for nurses of color, the fallout from speaking up can be more serious than for their white counterparts. Minority nurses are more reluctant to report incidents because they are more prone to be the victims of retaliation, especially if they are employed in low-minority healthcare settings. For example, in a mostly white environment, a black nurse reporting incidents or administrative problems is literally upsetting the apple cart. There is a price to pay, which sometimes is far too expensive for the nurse in question. Nurses from certain cultural backgrounds, such as Asians, Filipinos and Africans may be more reluctant to tattle, because they have been raised to respect authority and hierarchy. The cultural tradition is that you do not say anything, just remain quiet.

On a cautionary note, such behavior can be a Catch 22, "If you do not speak up, information gets distorted, and by the time you become involved, you will be the one written up for failing to report the incident. The resultant price can be extremely costly, but nevertheless, it is important that nurses of color do stand up for what is right thereby showing true professional integrity. Many nurses feel they have the support of their colleagues when discussing topics in private, but few feel openly supported by them.

It is apparent that nurses have never learned the true meaning of collegiality. However, in the words of Dr. Martin Luther King, I can proudly proclaim that "I have a dream—that one day nurses will have a mentally and emotionally safe environment in which to give caring and compassionate care. I have a dream that nurses will treat other nurses in ways that will not make members of the same profession feel diminished in any way, shape, or form." I have a dream, and I do want it to remain a dream, not a recurring nightmare.

While on night duty at a leading Montreal hospital, the nurse fell asleep, leaving the patients unattended for an undetermined period of her unauthorized somnolence. Sadly, during this grossly unacceptable lapse, an elderly female patient expired, and in a desperate bid to cover up the obvious neglect, the nurse decided to engage in what can be termed **"damage control"**. This was done by falsifying the clinical notes, to alter the time that the patient was last visited and turned, as well as the vital signs data. In some health care facilities, nodding off during break time while on the unit can be considered grounds for disciplinary action, the expectation being that nurses should be alert and available at any time. But she was also guilty of breaching the most fundamental tenet of the nursing profession by falsifying records. Trust had always been, and still is, the bedrock of the nursing profession, and these actions, by extension, succinctly bore traces of a lack of regard and respect for her peers.

It was a busy Saturday night on the Midwifery Unit at Mary Queen of Angels Hospital. We were slightly short- staffed as had become the norm on week-ends. In the obstetrical scenario, nurses have to remain calm, act fast, and carry out tasks. There were eight mothers in the Delivery Room, all in labor, some more advanced than others.

Unit routine dictates that for the first few hours following delivery, close monitoring of the vital signs of the newborn is essential and critical. In some cases labor has been lengthy and difficult, and as a result the baby could go "sour" in minutes.

I was responsible for the initial baths, placing them under radiant warmers to regulate their body temperature following the bath, administering routine newborn medications (Vitamin K), assisting in ensuring a proper latch during breast-feeding, ensuring that the baby was sucking well and getting adequate nutrition. I also answered the questions of the new mothers and, believe me, there were many, some of which seem to be asked only to appear intelligent in the eyes of the nurse.

I truly enjoyed my job and was happy all the time, but confessedly there were moments when second thoughts were being entertained. One night, the silence of the Unit was broken by the shrill voice of a middle aged-woman, whom I recognized as being the relative of one of our just-arrived new admissions.

"Oh, you have such a great job, you are so lucky," she said. "In fact, I am envious."

This remark immediately invoked my ire, although I did my utmost best to ensure that no sign of such an expression was visible on my face. It was certainly not the first time that my auditory canal had been subjected to such basic buccal vaporings. In essence and actuality, what she was really saying is that nurses do nothing except sit around during their shifts, cuddling and looking into the faces of newborns.

She had overlooked one vital fact—eight babies lined up in eight cribs, and two nurses with a pair of hands each I usually get an adrenaline rush, or (more aptly put), a high of sorts, on seeing first-time mothers cuddling their babies in a loving embrace, and the glimmer and sparkle in their eyes as they stare fixedly into the faces of their newborn.

Beside the happy veneer of the unit, lies another side. A call was received one hectic afternoon, from the Social Services Department, notifying us of their imminent arrival to pick up Baby John Doe for placement. He had been separated from his mother shortly after birth, and occupied a special place in the nursery. As he was prepared for departure, in unison the other nurses voiced their sadness at seeing him go, but all hoped that a bright future lay ahead of him.

It was not my place to judge, but so often I would hear a colleague comforting a crying baby quietly and indistinctly muttering, "I would cry, too, if I were you, and I was going home with them." Nonetheless,

I was certain that although some mothers were visibly incapable of caring for their newborns, they still carried a deep love within.

Historically, nurses have been categorized by certain stereotypes. They are supposed to be caring angels of mercy, an image created with the help of Florence Nightingale. Somewhere along the line, the angels of mercy moniker became attached to nurses as a group. While doctors display empathy, nurses administer boundless compassion and care. Regrettably, not all nurses are angels, and family members and doctors have repeatedly complained about some of the not-so-angelic angels.

The complaints have focused mostly on bad attitudes, use of uncouth language, and display of poor nursing ethics. Poor standards of nursing care, either by commission or omission, can also lead to complications. I have worked alongside so many nurses who did not possess a good grasp of the overall conditions of their patients, and who displayed little initiative to delve further, or widen their knowledge base. In the Pediatric Intensive Care Unit of Baby Care Hospital, Jean, a senior nurse who had worked over 18 years on the Unit, reported that 10 month old Baby Franklin, had been admitted with vocal cord paralysis and broncho-pulmonary disorder. The nurse's notes stated that Baby Franklin was seen awake, responsive, and smiling in his crib at 11:30 a.m. But a respiratory therapist had charted a change in Franklin's condition at 11:13 a.m.: "The infant is changing color. Respiratory distress is present. I have assessed him and he has a faint pulse."

At 11:46 a.m. the respiratory therapist was heard shouting for help, as Franklin was pale and in respiratory distress. Evidenced by nasal flaring, a "Code Blue" emergency was declared, but Franklin was pronounced dead despite the combined efforts of the medical staff, pediatricians, and cardiac team.

Yet another incident was reported to me by a mother, following the demise of her only son Devon while an in-patient at Turfbrooke General Hospital situated in the eastern part of England. The mother reported arriving early at the hospital to visit her son and happily was present for the rounds being conducted by the medical team.

She recalled, "I overheard two nurses talking in the corridor, just a few yards away from the entrance to my son's room. Walking slowly in their direction, she inquired, "Is there something wrong with my son, he doesn't look right.' One of the nurses said, "He had a good night! There's nothing wrong with him, for he just had breakfast and chatted with us". The nurses continued handing over the end of shift report, again the mother interrupted and in a pleading voice said, "He's not right" Mumbling under her breath, one of the nurses dismissively said to the mother, "The nurse has already told you he had a good night", whereupon she stood up and strode out of the Nursing Station.

On returning to her son's room the mother immediately noticed that her son had not been given his scheduled medication, since the pills were still in the medication cup on his bedside table. Devon's room was the next to be visited by the treating physician, who took one look at Devon, then started calling out to everyone, "Get in here quickly." There was a flurry of activity, including followed by the mother being politely ordered out of the room. About ten or more minutes later, she stood in the corridor and looked on in a somewhat befuddled gaze, as the slow exodus from the room began.

As the doctor slowly walked towards where she was standing, she knew the worst had occurred, and on entering the room following the brief exchange, seeing her son's body draped with a sheet, confirmation was established.

Warren, a 30 years old male, was admitted from home to the Emergency Department of Ladbrooke Hospital. He was intellectually challenged, with very limited speech, but enough to make his needs understood by his family. When Warren was admitted and showing signs of distress, the treating physician was called and visited on three occasions. On each occasion, his parents asked the doctor if there was anything wrong with his appendix or whether he had a bowel blockage. At that point in time, the doctor did not consider there was any cause for alarm. The parents were told that Warren had a virus, no name specified, and that his health was not in jeopardy. A few days later Warren began experiencing trouble sleeping, difficulty swallowing, followed by the onset of seizures. Clearly, he was now in severe distress. Warren's parents confessed that they had never seen him look so ill. Something was very seriously wrong, and again they inquired about his appendix and the possibility of a bowel blockage. Once more they were reassured that their son had a virus, and there was absolutely no cause for concern. Following a quick assessment, the Resident prescribed Paracetamol (Panadol) and Diazepam (Valium) to diminish the recurrence of his seizures. Both were to be administered in liquid form.

In the evening his condition worsened, and his parents voiced the same concern and repeated the earlier- asked question, only to receive the same response -- that he had a virus, except this time around an X-ray of the stomach was ordered by the doctor. Despite the medication adjustment and the requesting of specialized tests, the doctor continued to give the parents the impression that nothing was wrong with their son. Concomitantly, the nurses caring for Warren did not feel that anything was seriously wrong with him, and his uncommunicative state did little, if anything, to assist the situation. The parents also felt that certain members of staff displayed somewhat of a negative attitude towards their son because of his physical state and linguistic difficulty.

During the X-ray, Warren's mother noticed that his color was changing, she immediately alerted the technician, who realized that Warren had stopped breathing. A code was called and he was resuscitated, and transferred to the Coronary Intensive Care Unit. Death followed within two hours of his transfer. Cause of death was listed as peritonitis following perforation of his appendix, and paralytic ileus. Unable to verbally communicate, yet the medical and nursing staff failed to listen to the parents who knew him best, and who could have provided vital information about his condition.

# CHAPTER 9
# DEVOTION AND OBEDIENCE

> "No man, not even a doctor, ever gives any other definition of what a nurse should be than these – devoted and obedient."
>
> — *Florence Nightingale*

"**A** nurse must begin her work with the idea firmly implanted in her mind that she is only the instrument by whom the doctor gets his instructions carried out; she occupies no independent position in the treatment of the sick person" (McGregor-Robertson, 1902).

"No matter how gifted she may be, she will never become a reliable nurse until she can obey without question. The first and most helpful criticism I ever received from a doctor was that I was simply an intelligent machine for carrying out his orders". (*Dock, 1917*).

Things have certainly progressed since the above descriptions were prevalent. Nevertheless, many issues that affect how doctors and nurses work alongside each other stem from this traditional association. There are few professions where cooperation is as necessary as that between doctor and nurse. Yet, this traditional partnership has not been what it ought to be. I have seen failure to communicate effectively, and fundamental differences in the perception of the nurse's role.

The health care culture has permitted a certain degree of disrespect while considering this a normal style of communication. Doctors can at times be rude and uncouth, without a molecule of reservation. "Why are you calling me?" or "We'll get to it when we get to it," or "That's not important" all of which are undermining and disheartening serving as forces that impede functional doctor-nurse communication

The physician-nurse relationship can be stressful. The disciplines of nursing and medicine should interact for the health and well-being of the patients. While doctors and nurses appear to work harmoniously together, this apparently serene state of affairs is actually hiding inequality. Nurses need room to shine in the working environment, the traditional role of the doctor as the dominant professional means nurses face both structural and professional inequalities.

It is essential that nurses and doctors are able to exchange information in a coherent, comprehensive way. While doctors and nurses have individual, essential and specific roles within health systems, much recent work on patient safety and effective care points to a growing interdependence between these groups of professionals Garling (2008). Iedema (2009) goes as far as stating that communication is constitutive of healthcare, without communication, healthcare would not happen.

In every interaction with physicians, nurses have to prove their competence, while it is assumed that doctors are competent, and it is their fallibility and shortcomings that must be proven. Regardless of this inequality, nurses and doctors are required to work together towards a common goal. For in everyday practice, experienced nurses are usually the ones who induct and guide inexperienced junior doctors into the essential aspects of their disciplines. The relationship between doctor and nurse is to a large extent affected by what the patients think of them (Radcliffe, 2000).

Historically, becoming a good nurse has been equated with the fulfillment of doctors' wishes and instructions and capitulating, but today nurses are no longer playing the game. The truth be told, nurses are not playing any game. Behind the doctors' backs, nurses express resentment and act out their feelings. Some become "silent saboteurs," undermining or sabotaging, in a passive-aggressive way, decisions made by the medical team. Throughout my nursing career I have witnessed more times than I care to recall how nurses have visible difficulty in voicing their concerns or opinions regarding a member of the medical team, but conversely, with unmatched rapidity she would upbraid or denigrate a peer if she felt that she had committed a wrong.

Nurses are constantly faced with the task of having to call physicians requesting clarification or instruction in how to proceed in the care of a particular patient. Not always are doctors receptive to these calls. There are times when physicians have been known to become exasperatingly impatient when the inquiring nurse fails to have at hand all the pertinent information about the patient- a necessary requirement if the physician is to make a guided decision regarding the patient and the necessary treatment. Working in Canada and the U.S.A., I have witnessed situations where doctors have been verbally (or even somewhat physically) abusive toward nurses, shouting, or more aptly described, screaming) and, on one occasion, overheard publicly correcting them in language that was hugely derogatory of women and nurses.

A doctor might become frustrated with a new nurse who in his estimation demonstrates an inability to perform a task efficiently, or quickly enough. The workload of doctors compounded with time constraints could be an underlying cause of this impatience. There are doctors who get away with this display of professional misconduct, mainly because most nurses feel intimidated and avoid the risk of escalating the situation for fear of being disbelieved or discredited. Consequently, the behavior continues unchecked. After all, he is the doctor. In the eyes of the Administration, the doctor can do no wrong. Yes, nurses have continued (even up to present time) to do their darndest to cope with rude, unpleasant, dismissive, belittling, or downright intimidating physicians.

As a junior Staff Nurse, and many years later in the capacity of senior qualified Administrative Personnel, I recall speaking at a leadership session attended by Head Nurses, Charge Nurses, and even Departmental Heads about the unacceptable behavior of certain doctors, only to have my statements quickly dismissed with the following words: "Never mind, his bark is worse than his bite." "You must have misunderstood him, he has a soft heart". Or on the odd occasion, a puzzling look followed by, "That's strange, he is never like that".

I fail to recall any occasion, wherein a complaint verbal, written, or expressed concern regarding a physician or any member of the medical team brought by a nurse ever reached fruition, or at minimum a feedback beyond acknowledgement of receipt of the complaint.

Similarly, there are also physicians who will conveniently cast the blame on a nurse. A classic example to bear out this point is the doctor who reacts rudely to middle-of-the-night calls, although officially he is on call, and legally, the nurse must obtain his signature even for something as over-the-counter as Maalox or Tylenol. Once a nurse was heard commenting thus, "Most nurses are afraid to call Dr. X when they need to, and frequently won't."

Nurses see a strong association between disruptive physician behavior and adverse events, poor patient outcomes, and errors. Following is my description of the ward conduct, bedside manner and professional decorum of certain adherents of the Hippocratic Oath.

The doctor in question would come to the Unit, grab the chart of his patients, flip through a few pages with visible disinterest; ask no questions regarding nursing care, any changes in vital signs data, or untoward occurrence. Then he would quickly check the patient, write orders or reorders, and soon beat a hasty retreat. This doctor-patient-chart interaction or reaction takes less than five minutes in totality from start to finish. Through it all there has been no exchange of communication between medical and nursing staff.

Nurses including myself have stood by watching and waiting to either tell him about a particular patient, or for him to notify regarding a change in treatment. Oftentimes nurses have had to resort to eliciting responses from patients to ascertain the arrival or departure of this doctor. At other times the only giveaway of his presence was the disorganized clutter of charts sitting on the desk instead of being in their usual place on the rack. Despite having worked with this doctor for several years, he failed to address me by my name, resorting instead to the appellation "Nurse." It was blatantly apparent that no one seemed unduly concerned about the work ethic of this doctor. That was the accepted order of things in the work environment! Like so many others, I became an unwilling participant in the game of continued tolerance and silence.

Poor communication will continue as long as doctors view their roles and functions as fundamentally superior to those of nurses. Collaboration between physicians and nurses is rewarding when responsibility for patients' well-being is shared, as physicians and nurses do bring different perspectives to patient care. Nurses entering the workforce today are prepared for clinical independence, critical thinking, and professionalism. No longer do they view themselves as doctors' "handmaidens". Nor are they substitute doctors in general practice – they merely meet the needs of patients by approaching problems in a different way.

Before leaving the topic following situation indicates how Dr. Premmie, a third year resident in Pediatrics on a Neonatal Unit at Mary the Saint Hospital, came to realize how nurses are invaluable members of the healthcare team.

"I had been up the greater part of the night, having been on call. The next morning I was making the rounds and visiting some very ill babies, including one that had been 'Code Pink' some hours earlier," he explained. "I wrote an order in the baby's chart for an antibiotic, but due to increasing tiredness I put the decimal point in the wrong place, and if the nursing staff had not noticed and had given what I had ordered, we would have either lost that poor baby or caused severe damage to the kidneys and other organs". "Not to mention a likely lawsuit and loss of license to practice. I am so grateful to that nurse. At times I shudder to think what could have happened."

"I will forever remain grateful to her, and never forget how her knowledge and experience saved the day".

On realizing the mistake the Unit nurse immediately queried it and notified Dr. Premmie who immediately corrected the order.

It is not very often that nurses are at the receiving end of encomiums such as those verbalized by Dr. Premmie. The Head of the Medical Department once said to me in confidence, "I'm a doctor. We get all the glory and credit. And guess what? We only deserve part of it." Doctors will see patients anywhere from five to thirty minutes a day, and the rest of the time it is all nurses. They are the ones whom the patient first encounters, and their findings set us on the path towards a treatment and/or diagnosis confirmation. They are the ones making sure that patients get their pills and also check that vital signs are not dropping. They make sure that patients do not fall down and break any body part. When patients start vomiting, doctors run out but nurses stay and help".

In the book *Kill as Few Patients as Possible* the author Oscar London, M.D., sums it up: carefully and truthfully "Working with a good nurse is one of the great joys of being a doctor. I cannot understand physicians who adopt an adversarial relationship with nurses. They are depriving themselves of an education in hospital wisdom" (London, 2008. p.58).

A departmental discussion centered on an incident that had taken place on the Unit several weeks earlier. A senior nurse had approached a young intern, who at the time, had only been a few months out of medical school, and after voicing her concerns, requested that he listen to the heart rate of a particular patient. She had recently carried out auscultation, and had found it to be abnormally rapid. Without any visible effort to turn away from the chart and glance in her direction, his immediate brusque response was, "I do not need to, because I have seen the EKG." Thereupon he ended his retort. The nurse, true to her caring

79

nature, did not accept his response. She had a gnawing feeling that not only did she need to take further action, but also very soon.

She once again approached the intern and in a quiet, but firm voice, inquired if it was possible to see him away from the Nursing Station. He politely assented, and stood up to leave the area. Once together she explained to him that listening to the heart (auscultation) and an ECG report were not the same. While they both were focused on the same object, each had a different part of the story to tell. In the last twenty-four hours, the patient had seemingly developed a loud murmur and rapid heart rate. The intern appeared surprised at this new revelation, but nonetheless willingly carried out the nurse's request. Thankfully, this was done, for the patient was later transferred to the I.C.U with a diagnosis of early cardiac crisis.

No one could have sung the praises of that nurse any louder than the intern. In fact, he even hinted that she would make a good doctor and should strongly consider going to medical school. In this era of seeming communicative dysfunction, there are still some doctors who appreciate nurses, even those who point out their mistakes.

# CHAPTER 10
# PAPERWORK

> "Surely ghosts will follow wherever there is bad record keeping."
> — *Collin Dickey*

Nurses bear a large burden in managing and implementing the patient care plan of the interdisciplinary team, as well as documentation of progress made towards attaining these goals. Strange but true, most nurses routinely spend 20-25% of any average workday documenting patient care and in some cases considerably more time. This is not to be viewed as an issue per se, except that the perception held by most nurses is that much of this documentation is unnecessary or redundant. Above all, it detracts from their ability to administer direct patient care.

Throughout my career, from time to time nurses have repeatedly complained about the excessive burden of documentation, even citing it among the leading sources of dissatisfaction in their practice. Additionally, the issue has emerged in staff meetings and focus group discussions, with amassed evidence indicating that the increasing amount of time that nurses spend on documentation could be more appropriately spent on direct patient care.

Even up to and including my pre-retirement period, most of the overtime hours claimed by staff, irrespective of the shift worked, were attributed to time spent in the documentation of patient care. Notwithstanding the fact that no study of this kind had ever been conducted by any of the hospitals where I had been employed. I discovered during my discussion and parlance with the nurses, that at times other reasons were proffered, but documentation remained the dominant and causal factor, for delay in leaving work on time. Nevertheless, the nurses had to be paid for the additional hours worked, for failure to do so would certainly herald the intervention of the union, an action that the Hospital Administration strove to avoid at all costs.

It has been alleged that the issue of excessive time spent on nursing documentation has been a contributory factor in the subsequent exodus of nurses from the profession. Nurses have argued that they did not join the profession primarily to master the art of charting or writing, nor do they fantasize about proper documentation. Nevertheless, documentation remains a crucial part of patient care, and in today's healthcare arena the nurse not only has a professional responsibility, but can also be held accountable to document patient data that accurately reflects the assessment, planning, intervention, and evaluation of the patient's condition. Documentation is always the starting point in cases of malpractice. Therefore, the best defense is a good documentation offense.

Nursing documentation is seldom an issue until a crisis of severe proportions arises. Then and only then is documentation examined thoroughly. This has been my experience, and one that will not easily leave my mind. I am still awaiting the day when doctors, residents, or even medical students will read the progress notes of patients, with the degree of severity and importance they merit. Conversely, nurses do tend to read the doctors' notes far more often than those of their colleagues. Ultimately, it is the nurses' documentation that is expected to provide the most meaningful measure of the quality of care that has been delivered to the patient.

Even as nurses document, are they truly communicating? We have always been led to believe that nurses cannot make mistakes as they are dealing with lives. However, nurses are only humans, and like other humans they can make mistakes.

Some examples of documentation mistakes, otherwise known as **"CHARTING BLOOPERS"** committed by nurses.

**This is a 98 YO with a host of medical problems**

**Patient has no past history of suicides**

**The patient is actually a fairly reliable historian**

**Order: Discharge home when strong**

**Patient unresponsive but in no distress**

**Denies any rectal bleeding**

**Non-verbal, non-communicative and no problems**

**Patient is 95% blind.**

**Pussy eyes.**

**67-year-old female admitted following partial TAH.**

**Chief complaint—bazaar behavior.**

**Foley emptied for fowl smelling urine.**

**Patient walking unaccompanied in hell.**

**Fecal heart tones heard**

**Pt. observed to be seeping quietly.**

**Large BM walking in the hall**

**Large BM walking in the hall.**

**Patient had pelvic exam done on the floor.**

**Vaginal packing out. Doctor in.**

One mid-summer evening, a middle-aged patient was expected on the unit, having been transferred from a hospital in Northern Quebec. The nurse on the previous shift wrote in the chart and in the end of shift report: **"Patient expected late evening. Notify doctor immediately patient hits the floor."**

Breda, a nurse in the Maternal and Child Care Unit of Mary the Saint Hospital, was relaxing at home one evening when she received a telephone call from the Nursing Supervisor, requesting an explanation of nursing documentation while on the day shift. During the day she had assisted the obstetric Resident in carrying out a pelvic examination. Her entry read like this: **"Pelvic examination carried out by resident with nurse in lithotomy position."**

# CHAPTER 11
# GRATITUDE

> "I can no other answer make, but, thanks, thanks, and thanks."
>
> — *William Shakespeare*

T he evening shift in the psychiatric Unit at All Saints Hospital was extremely busy because of two nearly fatal suicide attempts during the earlier shift. I had just commenced my night shift, feeling somewhat overly tired due to an inadequate amount of sleep during the day. I tried my utmost best to complete my shift, giving the clock in the nurses' station a nod of approval with each passing hour.

In the early hours of the morning, the Charge Nurse informed me that I was mandated under "force majeures" to work an additional four hours, on account of a shortage of nurses on the day shift. Despite my being tired, in addition to having a previously- scheduled medical appointment later in the morning, I was told in no uncertain terms that the Charge Nurse was not making a request, but instead giving a directive. I had already worked twelve hours, forced to work another four, and to return for my next twelve hour shift with only a few hours between. I managed to survive the extra four forced hours, but they were the longest four hours that I can recall.

Leaving the Unit at the end of the shift, I was greeted by Mercy, one of my former mentors. She leaned over, grabbed me and gave me a warm supportive hug, "Thank you! Thank You! Thank You! she echoed. I was somewhat taken aback, and possessed no idea of the underlying reason(s) behind the expressed sentiments. Requesting an explanation she told me that she was extremely grateful that I had worked the extra hours, as she was unable to come in earlier due to an inability to find a replacement for her ill babysitter. I felt really appreciated and gave her a huge hug in return.

Time and time again, the question has been asked whether nurses get the recognition they truly deserve. Unequivocally, the answer is a resounding NO! We do not get enough respect from doctors or from administrators. But more importantly, we fail among ourselves to receive and give compliments or recognition to each other.

Some patients and their families go out of their way to show appreciation for all our hard work and compassion. Then there are others who give praise and thanks to the doctors, residents, and even the medical student, whom they encountered for only a fleeting moment, or a handful of minutes during their stay, compared to the nurses who were at the bedside round the clock. Yes, nurses should be recognized for the good work that they do, but I assert these feelings should come from within.

We need to celebrate each other's accomplishments. While nurses sometimes fumble and falter accepting praise, they are equally slow in offering it to a peer. During report time, we need to make sure that fellow nurses are complimented for procedures well carried out, swift action taken, or a crisis averted. In a direct and honestly truthful manner, a peer can be told how you felt about the tasks completed, the emergency averted etc. It can be as small as, "Wow, you did all that during your shift? "You must have been super busy", "I wonder if I could have done all that," "Thanks for being such an asset to our team".

Recognition helps build trust and create a positive work environment for the entire team.

During a Nurses Week celebration ceremony, where several nurses were being honored for outstanding practice and professionalism, the following scenario unfolded.

Following a brief introduction by the chief obstetrician and gynecologist, one of the awardees stepped up to the podium and said to the smiling audience, "Thanks, but I do not deserve this reward". Sadly, this attempt at modesty became self-deprecation. I understood what this nurse meant: she did not want to be singled out when she knew her fellow nurses did as equally good a job. However, both she and the profession would have been better served if she had responded in this manner, "I accept this award on behalf of my colleagues who do an outstanding job every day."

Being humble and gracious is one thing, but the undervaluation of one's self is another. Of course much of this is learned behavior since some were raised to believe that accepting praise or compliment is a sign of pride. Others have the misguided belief that acknowledging a compliment is a form of conceit. Conversely, if praise and compliments are routinely deflected a person appears to lack confidence and is unworthy of recognition.

In reconditioning our responses by learning to accept and give well-deserved praise and gratitude, we can lift ourselves and our profession to the higher level where they both belong.

# CHAPTER 12
# PERSPECTIVES

N urses are oftentimes asked why they chose their profession. As outlined earlier in this memoir, following the sudden unexpected demise of my younger sister, and seeing the way she was cared for it was an immediate decision that nursing would be my chosen career. Prior to my migration to commence my nursing career, I met some healthcare professionals (midwives and community nurses) who worked in my community. They served as further models of inspiration.

I decided to ask some of my colleagues the reason(s) behind their becoming a nurse. I was surprised by some of the responses and taken aback by a few.

Venus is a graduate nurse with three years' experience working in surgery.

*"Nursing was actually chosen for me, as it was a guidance counselor in high school that suggested this profession. She saw something in me that I did not see in myself, and suggested that I attend a Career Fair so that I could further explore my options. At that Fair I discovered that nurses save lives, were very well respected, and helped those that could not help themselves.*

*"I was hooked—what better way to live a life than to help others? Once I left high school, I went to college to pursue nursing studies.*

*"To be honest, today I cannot imagine doing anything other than nursing. However, before my high school guidance counselor suggested that I should go into nursing, I had actually thought of being an airline hostess and traveling the world. Through nursing, I have been able to make some part of the traveling dream come true".*

Lisa, a Registered Nurse trained in Western Canada, and who has worked in several parts of the United States.

*"I cannot really recall why I chose nursing, but I do know that it was not my first choice of a profession. I had previously worked in the bank as a teller, and later as a clerk in an accounting firm. I needed stable employment and as such I gravitated towards nursing. For me it was a viable option. It was certainly not my first choice, as I can clearly recall. Over the years I have grown to love nursing, and have clung fixedly to the age-old Hippocratic dictum: 'First do no harm.'*

*"I have been a wound nurse for quite some time, but while I still love hands-on care, I find the amount of documentation staggering. The administration expects you to do 15 hours of work in 12 hours, including documentation, and they yell about overtime when it happens. As much as I hate the amount of charting that is expected of each and every nurse, the real truth, as everyone knows, is this: 'If it isn't written, it wasn't done!' My reward comes when I look patients in the eye and see that they are grateful for my attention. For me it answers the question of why I became a nurse."*

Jasmine, an R.N employed in the Obstetrics Department of Mary Saints Hospital, graduated seven years ago.

*"My mother was a nurse, and I had two aunts who were also nurses, so the expectation during my teenage years was that I would also become a nurse. I grew up watching my mother put on her nursing uniform and cap for work and never really thought I would enter the profession. It*

*was as though I had no choice. In fact, I didn't. I was not even permitted the opportunity to think of any other job, not even for a moment, as my mother walked, talked, breathed, and even dreamed nursing. While I was still in elementary school, my mother referred to me as 'a nurse in the making.' She had already defined my life's goals that early, seemingly even before my cranium had reached full development. I carried this imposed burden all the way through college, not wanting to disappoint my mother, finally allowing her lifelong desires to reach fruition in my becoming a registered nurse.*

*"Personally, I cannot share the same feelings as my mother, for I am tired of 'running a marathon' each evening at work. But I love the moments when a patient thanks me and says they are getting such good care. It makes my day, and keeps me going into each room with a smile and positive outlook. I feel good that I became a nurse, for there is no other profession where so many people can thank you at any time. That keeps me going and reminds me of what nursing is all about."*

Lee-Anne, a recent graduate, pursued a baccalaureate degree at an on-line university.

*"I became a nurse due to my being hooked on Gray's Anatomy and E.R. Yes, I was raised in the era of television. However, my desire was not merely to help others and all that smoochy stuff. Certainly not! I liked the glamour of the E.R, the adrenalin rush, and most of all mixing with all the interns and their supervisors. You can literally say that I glamorized nursing, as my view did not include bedpans, urinals, colostomies, feces, emesis, wet beds, etc. No way! No day! To compound matters I had no friends who were nurses, so there was no one to ask what the profession really entailed. Plainly put, I was in my own world and quite enjoying it.*

*"While I am trying my best to enjoy the profession, I hate the term 'just a nurse.' What does that really mean? I am not 'just a nurse.' Over the course of eight hours, I can interpret blood gases, monitor vital signs, administer medications, and comfort a dying patient. So the term 'just*

*a nurse' is inept. I may not be a doctor, but I am a nurse, not 'just a nurse.' A doctor does not have to be distinguished in terms of his workload or work performance. He remains a doctor. I did not become a nurse because I could not pass the grade in medical school. I love what I do. I am a nurse and always will be."*

Nursing is a profession and a lifestyle. It guides us how we choose to live our own lives and how we influence the lives of all those around us. It is a powerful profession that allows us the opportunity to bring people into the world, and to be there with people when they depart this life. It allows us the opportunity to support those in grief and to join in the celebration of recovery. I like to think of my nursing career as a journey, on an adventurous route, with challenging experiences, and an ever-present fear of the unknown. For me, it has certainly been a truly fantastic journey. I have no regrets. Today, not many nurses talk about the profession with the passion and joy that it truly merits.

Lazarus, Second career male nurse, employed in the psychiatric department of All Saints Hospital.

*"Being raised as a Catholic and also being Italian, my mother was very excited regarding my choice of profession. She strongly felt that this was in line with the teachings of our religion. Dad, however, was not as excited, and it took some time before he finally came around to accepting my choice. I had thought of nursing while pursuing my first degree, but thought it was inappropriate because I didn't know any nurses who were men. I knew there were names being tossed around regarding male representatives of the nursing profession.*

*I was seriously considering my career options and from time to time nursing came to the forefront. I decided to invest some time in soliciting advice from some of my friends' parents who were nurses. The consensus of the advice that I received was that I should firstly become a nursing assistant to see if that was what I really wanted to do. If so, then I could proceed to further training toward my nursing registration. Great, I thought! I started working as a part-time nurse's aide on a medical unit doing the night shift. I learned so much and felt like this would be a career, not just another job. For me it was truly a humbling but enriching experience.*

*For a man in a female-dominated profession, issues of authority are expressed differently. Sometimes it seems there are less flexibility and a greater black and white perspective in this realm. I found myself keeping a low profile in my work roles because some of the women seemed uncomfortable working with a man. Being introduced as a male student nurse on a Labour and Delivery Unit does not exactly provide a yellow brick road when first meeting a female patient and tact and professionalism are required when interacting with the patient. Surprisingly, I have found that many patients simply assume that I'm a doctor. I become equally frustrated when asked why I'm 'just a nurse' and didn't remain in school a few extra years and become a doctor.*

*"Despite the complexity of the work environment, I now recognize how well these components blend. With my passion for people, I sometimes think that nursing chose me."*

After many years as a nurse, I can most concisely add my own perspective to the discussion by offering the following lists (which confessedly may be woefully incomplete).

# WHAT I HAVE LEARNED ABOUT NURSING

1. Saying that I am a nurse is entirely different from being a nurse.
2. Patients will teach me more about nursing than I will ever teach them.
3. Some patients are in our lives for only a short while, but we are often in theirs for the rest of it.
4. The very first medication a nurse gives is a dose of reality; her second dose is humility.
5. Nursing is still among the most respected occupations, despite nurses being regularly discredited and abused.

6. A nurse has to wear many faces for many cases: a carer, a sharer, a boulder, a shoulder to lean or cry on, a healer, a sealer, a dealer, a feeler, a teacher, a reacher, a preacher, a marathon walker, a protector, a detector, a mathematician, a diagnostician, a friend to the end.

# WHAT I WILL MISS ABOUT NURSING

1. The honor of being involved with patients in their most vulnerable state.
2. The instant trust that patient places in you merely because you were assigned to care for them.
3. The enlightening conversations about personal, religious and moral values that I have participated in with patients.
4. The care I gave to help a patient progress from hopeless to hopeful.
5. The bitter-sweet effect of being telephoned and asked to stay at home due to low census.
6. The sense of accomplishment that accompanies the completion of a particularly difficult nursing task, such as a successful I.V insertion on a patient with difficult veins, or a complex dressing change.
7. Working with doctors and helping to find solutions and remedies for patients' problems and concerns.
8. Being totally impressed with the teamwork displayed by the healthcare team during any CODE (BLUE OR PINK).

# WHAT I WILL NOT MISS ABOUT NURSING

1. Leaving home at 6.30 p.m., ready for my twelve- hour night shift I will certainly not miss.
2. Planning dinners, parties, family events, and birthday celebrations around my weekend and holiday work schedule.
3. The hospital policy: "I can be sick for as long as I am actually sick."
4. CPR renewal days, especially when I was getting too old to spend half a day on the floor pressing down on plastic babies and adults with my whole upper body strength.

5. Holding my urine some nights until I no longer had the urge to go and then wondering: where it all went.
6. The night shift, which I did most of the time throughout my career. While I absolutely loved the night staff, I could not always remember how I got home in the morning.
7. The uncertainty of vacation period (seniority).
8. Xmas off only if ill or high seniority status.

# GOALS FOR IMPROVEMENT

## 1. Elimination of Lateral Hostility

As a profession we will continue to hold ourselves back until we are united, stand strong together and pledge to eliminate the horrendous act of "nurses eating their young". We must eliminate the well- known cattiness and the bullying that so often is encountered by new nurses. After all, we are an integral part of a beautiful and caring profession. Hence, let us extend and demonstrate that care to our fellow nurses as well as our patients.

## 2. Treat every patient encounter as an Educational Opportunity

Every encounter with the patient should be taken as an opportunity to educate. It can be about their condition, treatment they are receiving, their medication, their hospital stay or a procedure they are receiving, with attention to details. Always ask patients if they have any questions, and take the time to answer thoughtfully and responsibly. Patients are appreciative of the extra time a nurse may spend giving them extra attention, and they may not always ask the questions they need to.

## 3. Continue to grow professionally and personally through Continuing Education

Regardless of the employers' requirements, nurses need to take personal responsibility for continuing their education. This does not infer being in college until death intervenes, or the pursuance of higher degree. What it does mean is that healthcare and nursing are constantly evolving, and you should be aware of advances that will help you provide the best care possible for your patients. This may include reading nursing articles and blogs, looking for evidence- based practice, and other sources of information. Anything that expands your knowledge base as a nurse is helpful in helping your growth. It should be noted, however, that if you intend to use your knowledge to change your practice, or the organization you work for, you should ensure that the information is vetted and evidence- based.

## 4. Encourage more males to join the profession

Male nurses (Murses) constitute a fraction of our profession. However, they do bring a unique perspective to nursing, and we should be thrilled with every Y chromosome that is added to our ranks. Encourage your male friends and family to pursue a nursing career, for having more men in the nursing profession is a great benefit.

## 5. Mandate a safe staffing ratio

Already many hospitals throughout the United States have implemented nurse patient ratios to promote safety and improve care. However, this is not universal. Canada has yet to make a move in this direction. Until this becomes a requirement, there will be too many opportunities for nurses to have unsafe patient loads and risk not being able to provide safe and competent care.

# CHAPTER 13
# AND MIGHT I ADD

"Life does not cease to be funny when someone dies any more than it ceases to be serious when people laugh."

— *George Bernard Shaw*

Despite the popularity of humor therapy, this treatment modality has not gained wide acceptance in mainstream medicine. I have found this to be true throughout my nursing career. Laughter is well known for its healing properties. Even a two-minute titter releases enough feel-good chemicals (endorphins) to cheer up a gloom-fogged brain. It also lowers levels of the stress hormones adrenaline and cortisol, and clears stale air from the lungs. A true full-on belly laugh can also burn excess calories and leave us with a euphoric "afterglow" in which we relax tense muscles.

There has been endless talk by experts, especially psychologists, about effective coping strategies and their impact on an individual's mental and physical health. I am not suggesting clowns squirting water at seriously ill patients, or slipping whoopee cushions under people recuperating from bowel surgery. Perhaps a "mirth menu" from which patients could choose the most effective recovery diet. The infusion of humor into our daily routines makes perfect sense to keep staff happy. They will become more enthusiastic and less prone to hide in the bathroom, or take extended coffee breaks. My personal defense against the nuances of life has always been my sense of humor—whether it is imagining the not-so-nice supervisor being chased naked by an angry dog or playing a practical joke on the know-it-all resident.

I do share some concern that patients will perceive nurses as being unprofessional and unconcerned about their health problems if they show a sense of humor while interacting with them. Of course, the nurse should determine a patient's humor preference, and state of mind before cracking a well-intended but ill-timed joke, causing the patient some degree of mental anguish and the nurse to be unappreciated. Concerning the last point I speak from the pulpit of personal experience.

While pursuing Part 1 Midwifery studies in Birmingham, England, at a hospital well- renowned for its highly specialized Premature Baby Unit, I conducted an unassisted vaginal delivery. The patient was a young primigravida, who had undergone an uncomplicated but lengthy first stage of labour. Following a successful delivery, and clamping of the umbilical cord the baby was handed over to the mother. Shortly thereafter as was the protocol, the baby was then taken out of the Delivery Room to be administered routine post-delivery care. While we awaited the delivery of the placenta, which heralded the completion of the third and final stage of labour, the mother, tired but overjoyed, soon engaged me in a conversation that went like this:

**Patient:** "Nurse, how is baby doing? Is she all right? Is she okay?"

**Nurse:** "Yes, she looks fine on the outside. Don't know what's happening on the inside."

**Patient:** "Oh!"

There was no further verbal interaction between us. The patient was later transferred to the Post-Partum Unit, following a satisfactory examination and assessment. A few days later, a very serious Head Nurse summoned me to her office, requesting to know what had taken place between me and this particular patient, following delivery. Apparently following her transfer to the unit, the patient was extremely tearful and displaying signs of anxiety, to the point that she refused to eat and drink. She had made repeated requests to see the pediatrician, claiming that the nurse who had delivered her baby had said that something was wrong with the baby's stomach and intestines. She kept the baby in her arms at all times, refusing to put it in its crib for fear that it would vomit and aspirate, or that it would need surgery for the non-functioning bowel and intestines.

In hushed but sincere tones, I carefully explained verbatim what I had said to the mother following the delivery. I explained to the Head Nurse that humor was intended when I replied I could only see the outside and not the inside. Ironically, as I was recounting there was a strange and insensitive ring to it. I now realized how tactless and uncaring, not to mention unprofessional my remarks had sounded, especially to a recently delivered first-time parent. I was learning firsthand about the mental and emotional fragility of postpartum patients.

The Head Nurse paused for what to me seemed like eternity, and then slowly walked away from her desk and gently placed her hands on my left shoulder. I am certain that my entire body had taken on an ashen-gray hue, as I felt as if the blood was leaving my body. My career was on the verge of coming to a sad and abrupt close, or so I thought.

She looked me in the face and sternly said, "British humor is not the same as in other countries." She then paused, as if searching for the right words to say, and then continued, all the while still holding my shoulder: "What may be seen as a joke for you, may be stress for another person. Keep jokes out of your work."

I waited to ensure that she had finished her speech, and, with my eyes cast to the floor, I apologized for my seemingly blatant and uncaring attitude, faithfully promising that there would be no recurrence of such an incident. I felt my heart pounding, and my knees felt as if they would give way under me if I did not assume a sedentary position soon. I had initially feared the worst, and now I was silently grateful for the outcome. I needed a place of safety, where I could allow my heart an opportunity to resume its normal rhythm.

From that moment onwards, I clung firmly to an old adage, and one that I will always remember: "Easy lessons are good for dunces, and tough schools are for fools." I was neither a dunce nor a fool, so that the school or the learning would no longer be applicable to me. At least I didn't think so. I had been warned and intended to govern myself accordingly and professionally.

In the day to day working environment there is always someone or something that serves as a mental irritant, even as far removed as the clerk in the payroll office or the dietician in the dietary department. The irritant may also be close to home as the colleague who fails to pull her weight.

Identified below are some of the common unit personalities, there is usually two or more on any unit in any hospital.

## PHONE DRONE

No one wants to hear about the quarrel you had with your husband or live-in mate last night. Factor me out of your weekend country cottage plans, or the embarrassing thing your neighbor did at the weekend barbecue. Forgive me if this sounds uncaring and insensitive, but no one wants to hear about your kids' shots and the bad night they had post-inoculation. Even innocuous subjects should rarely be discussed at length on the phone within earshot of patients and nurses. Personal conversations can make your peers very uncomfortable, and constant chatting on the phone, especially about non-hospital topics, can make you look like someone who's not getting work done. Wait until the shift is over before making personal phone calls. The hospital phone is for work-related conversations only. Put your cell phone away also, the Utility Room is not for your utilization.

## UNTIDY HEIDI

Soda cans, coffee cups, alcohol swabs, crumpled Kleenexes, medical supplies, and even leftover food—we have all seen these things pile up,

Andean high, in the Nursing Lounge. You may be saying to yourself that it doesn't harm anyone. It bothers people more than you think. If your locker is so cluttered that your mess infringes on another nurse's space, it will attract fruit flies and may also soil important documents. You will soon earn yourself the reputation of being sloppy, immature, and incompetent—not a great trio of characteristics!

Cleanliness is important in the hospital, and that applies to your space, too.

## THE SNACKING NURSE

This nurse is always snacking, munching on a candy bar, a carrot, chomping away on an apple or holding a diet beverage.

## MISSING IN ACTION—FAR FROM THE WAR

While everyone else is busy on the unit looking after patients, charting, or dealing with family matters, you are nowhere to be found. Lost in space or out of the race? You are either taking a prolonged lunch, one of your many self-assigned breaks, or have called in sick (again). While nobody wants to see you chained to your routine, leaving your patients untended and your doctor uninformed makes you seem lazy, and causes your colleagues to be forced to pick up your workload. You might think it's nobody's business, but that's the thing about work—everything is everyone else's business. We are a team. People are constantly comparing themselves to their peers and superiors alike, and will grow to resent people who don't seem to be putting in a full shift's work. Are you wondering if people notice how often you're outside talking on your cell phone or leaving before the end of your shift. Stop wondering and relax your cardio-respiratory system. They have noticed.

# BROWN NOSER

Even worse than the "far from the war" employee is the nurse who blatantly tries at every opportunity to outshine everyone else. She takes full credit for another nurse's work, throws a fellow nurse under the bus during a staff meeting, and constantly makes disingenuously flattering compliments to the nursing supervisor. While you may need to let those in authority know that you are performing well in your job, it is best to be discreet and let your skills and actions speak for themselves. Give credit to other nurses when and where it is due, and do not tattle on others unless necessary. Keep to a minimum any compliments regarding the color-coordinated apparel of the Head Nurse or Supervisor.

# CONSTANT COMPLAINER

Nurses do need to vent sometimes, but should always remember that work is called work for a reason. However, if you spend an inordinate amount of time airing grievances about the hospital or your life to anyone who will listen, you are certainly not going to succeed in making things better, especially if your grievances concern patients and hospital policies. Do not venture there. Just because the nurse or doctor you're complaining about doesn't say anything, it does not mean that he or she agrees with you. Wrong again on all counts! They're probably just hoping you'll stop complaining and leave the hospital soon.

# GABBY GOSSIP

You can always see them. When they are not at the front desk whispering to the secretary or Unit Coordinator, they are surreptitiously surfing sites looking for news of any sort. If anyone is having an affair, starting a pregnancy or getting fired, they are usually the first to know, whether or not that information is actually correct. No time for validation. Time for a word of caution and advice here—In the hospital environment, people always notice those who are in the middle of gossip. If you find yourself in secretive conversations with individuals known for having loose lips, you will be judged guilty by virtue of association. Those who assemble usually resemble.

# PRANKSTERS

Pranks around the hospital are appreciated only in small doses, and any involving patients are out of the question. There is a time and place for occasional pranks within the hospital environment; any more beyond that, and they become nightmarish. Even peers with a good sense of humor will quickly become tired of your antics. They will become annoyed if they cannot leave their desks for a moment without returning to mixed up patients' charts, misplaced medication sheets, or a computer that suddenly doesn't work. Just remember that if you do any of the aforementioned actions on a regular basis and see no problem with your actions, you may very well be the most annoying person in the hospital. The psychiatrist may soon come calling.

## THE DOUBLES NURSE

The Energizer Bunny has nothing on this nurse. She will work every extra shift available, be it day, evening or night, any season and for any reason. She will even brag about the number of hours that she has worked without a wink of sleep. She is working her way into the Guiness Book Of Records.

## THE NO- NONSENSE NURSE

This is the nurse who has earned credibility on the Unit., and a reputation as the nose-to-the- grindstone worker. In her presence all nurses straighten up and get on task. Everyone fears a cold stare or glare.

## THE SALES NURSE

She always has something to sell, and the items for sale are not all medical or nursing related. Household items are sometimes included. She will never disclose the source of her supply, and she is often unable to get you the same item again.

# THE IRREVERENT NURSE

This nurse is hilarious and lots of fun to be around. She usually says out loud what the majority of other nurses were thinking but were too timid to say. She is loud and outspoken, broadcasting that she does not care what anyone thinks of her.

# CHAPTER 14
# BACK TO THE FUTURE

"Tomorrow is a new day, you shall begin it with too high a spirit to be encumbered with your old nonsense."

— *Ralph Waldo Emerson*

More than ever nurses can make a positive impact on the lives of the patients they serve and their colleagues who will follow them. Nurses are on the frontline of healthcare but on the receiving end of budget cuts regulatory requirements. While the Administration may be planning the "how to", the nurses are the ones who really see the full effects. They are the active agents who deliver the product.

The healthcare industry faces unprecedented challenges, for it is also coping with the aging patient 'silver tsunami" effect. Greater life expectancy of individuals with chronic and acute conditions will challenge the ability of the healthcare system to provide efficient and effective continuing care. While there is no escaping the budget cuts that are associated with healthcare effects, there is some escape from the potential negative effects on the nursing profession. As nurses we must reach deep within ourselves and unearth the confidence to advocate for ourselves and the profession.

In the 21st century nurses must be skilled in the use of computer technology. This is imperative in a collaborative healthcare environment, many of which bear little to no resemblance to the hospital centric practice of yore. At the same time the new generation of nursing students is demanding information faster than instructors can deliver it by classroom methods.

The nursing curriculum needs to be adapted to satisfactorily equip this new generation of tech savvy learners. Advances in digital technology have increased the application of telehealth and telemedicine, bringing together patient and provider without physical proximity (Zhang, 2019). Nanotechnology will introduce new forms of clinical diagnosis and treatment by means of inexpensive handheld biosensors capable of detecting a wide range of diseases from miniscule body specimens. (Staggers, 2008).

Already distance learning modalities link students and faculties from different locations and expand the potential for accessible continuing professional education. The healthcare delivery system of the future will rely on teams of nurses, nurse practitioners, physicians, social workers and others to work together. Technically sophisticated preclinical simulation laboratories will stimulate critical thinking and skill acquisition in a safe and user-friendly environment. There will be a further growing need for interdisciplinary education for collaborative practice. Here a wide range of knowledge and skills is required to effectively and efficiently manage the comprehensive needs of patients and populations (Orey, 2010).

# CHAPTER 15
# HISTORY OF NURSING

> "Let us never consider ourselves finished nurses…we must be learning all of our lives."
>
> — *Florence Nightingale*

The word "nurse" originally came from the Latin word "nutrire", meaning to suckle, referring to a **wet-nurse**.; Only in the late 16th century did it attain its modern meaning of a person who cares for the infirm.

Beginning from the earliest times a stream of nurses dedicated to service on religious principles was produced by most cultures. Both Christendom and the Muslim World generated a stream of dedicated nurses from their earliest days. In Europe, before the foundation of modern nursing, Catholic nuns and the military often provided nursing-like services. Not until the 19th century did nursing become a secular profession. In the 20th century nursing became a major profession in all modern countries, and was a favored career for women.

Ashoka, Buddhist Indian ruler (268 BC to 232 BC) erected a series of pillars, which included an edict ordering hospitals to be built along the routes of travelers, and that they be "well provided with instruments and medicine, consisting of mineral and vegetable drugs, with roots and fruits"; "Whenever there is no provision of drugs, medical roots, and herbs, they are".

In **Romans 16:1** the first known Christian nurse, Phoebe, is mentioned. During the early years of the Christian Church (ca. AD 50), St. Paul sent a deaconess named Phoebe to Rome as the first visiting nurse. (De Witt, 2009). From its earliest days, following the edicts of Jesus, Christianity encouraged its devotees to tend the sick. Priests were often also physicians. while pagan religions seldom offered help to the infirm, the early Christians were willing to nurse the sick and take food to them, notably during the smallpox epidemic of AD 165-180 and the measles outbreak of around AD 250; In nursing the sick and dying, regardless of religion, the Christians won friends and sympathizers".

Following the First Council of Nicaea in AD 325, Christianity became the official religion of the Roman Empire, leading to an expansion of the provision of care. Among the earliest were those built ca. 370 by St. Basil the Great, bishop of Caesarea Mazaca in Cappadocia in Asia Minor (modern-day Turkey), by Saint Fabiola in Rome ca. 390, and by the physician-priest Saint Sampson (d. 530) in Constantinople, Called the Basiliad, St. Basil's hospital resembled a city, and included housing for doctors and nurses and separate buildings for various classes of patients. There was a separate section for lepers. Eventually, the construction of a hospital in every cathedral town was begun.

Christian emphasis on practical charity gave rise to the development of systematic nursing and hospitals after the end of the persecution of the early church. Ancient church leaders like St. Benedict of Nursia (480-547) emphasized medicine as an aid to the provision of hospitality.

12th century Roman Catholic orders like the Dominicans and Carmelites have long lived in religious communities that work for the care of the sick. (Stewart et al.,1962)

# MEDIAEVAL EUROPE

Medieval hospitals in Europe followed a similar pattern to the Byzantine. They were religious communities, with care provided by monks and nuns. (An old French term for hospital is *hôtel-Dieu*, "hostel of God.") Some were attached to monasteries; others were independent and had their own endowments, usually of property, which provided income for their support. Some hospitals were multi-functional while others were founded for specific purposes such as leper hospitals, or as refuges for the poor, or for pilgrims: not all cared for the sick. The first Spanish hospital, founded by the Catholic Visigoth bishop Masona in AD 580 at Mérida, was a ***xenodochium*** designed as an inn for travellers (mostly pilgrims to the shrine of Eulalia of Mérida) as well as a hospital for citizens and local farmers. The hospital's endowment consisted of farms to feed its patients and guests. From the account given by Paul the Deacon we learn that this hospital was supplied with physicians and nurses, whose mission included the care the sick wherever they were found, "slave or free, Christian or Jew." During the late 700s and early 800s, Emperor Charlemagne decreed that those hospitals which had been well conducted before his time and had fallen into decay should be restored in accordance with the needs of the time. He further ordered that a hospital should be attached to each cathedral and monastery.

In the West, everyone knows Florence Nightingale, in many ways the founder of modern nursing. However, many centuries earlier, a woman named Rufaida Al-Aslamia introduced nursing to the Muslim world. She is estimated to have been born in the year 620 — exactly 1,200 years before Florence Nightingale. Just like Florence Nightingale, who became famous when tending for the wounded during the Crimean War, it was war that brought Al-Aslamia to nursing. She learnt many medical skills by assisting her father, a famous healer, and converted to Islam after religion's "Holy Prophet", Muhammad, settled in her hometown of Medina. During the early battles of his followers, she provided first aid to injured soldiers, made sure they had drinking water, and arranged shelter from the heat and the desert wind for the wounded and dying. In similarity to Nightingale, who trained a team of volunteer nurses, Rufaida did not go alone, leading a group of Muslim women to work with her. At the end of the wars, Muhammad gave Rufaida permission to erect a tent inside the Prophet's Mosque (Al-Masjid an-Nabawi) in Madina to keep providing nursing care, and to train more Muslim women and girls as nurses. She advocated for preventative care and is even said to have drafted the world's first code of nursing conduct and ethics (Miller-Rosser et al, 2006)

During the tenth century the monasteries became a dominant factor in hospital work. The famous Benedictine Abbey of Cluny, founded in 910, set the example which was widely imitated throughout France and Germany

No less efficient was the work done by the diocesan clergy in accordance with the disciplinary enactments of the councils of Aachen (817, 836), which prescribed that a hospital should be maintained in connection with each collegiate church. The canons were obliged to contribute towards the support of the hospital.

When they conquered England in 1066, the Normans brought their hospital system along. Merging with traditional land-tenure and customs, the new charitable houses became popular and were distinct from both English monasteries and French hospitals. They dispensed alms and some medicine, and were generously endowed by the nobility and gentry who counted on them for spiritual rewards after death.

In France, rich families continued to fund convents and monasteries, and enrolled their daughters as nuns who provided free health services to the poor. Nursing was a religious role for the nurse, and there was little call for science (Jones, 1989).

The Crimean War was a significant development in nursing history when English nurse Florence Nightingale laid the foundations of professional nursing with the principles summarized in the book *Notes on Nursing*. Canadian nursing dates all the way back to 1639 in Quebec with the Augustine nuns, who came from Dieppe. In 1644, five years after their arrival, they founded the first permanent hospital in New France, the Hôtel-Dieu, exactly where the hospital is today. These nuns were trying to open up a mission that cared for the spiritual and physical needs of patients. The establishment of this mission created the first nursing apprenticeship training in North America. In 1874 the first formal nursing training program was started at the General and Marine Hospital in St. Catharines, Ontario, Canada.

## MIDDLE EAST

The Eastern Orthodox Church had established many hospitals in the Middle East, but following the rise of Islam from the 7th century, Arabic medicine developed in this region, where a number of important advances were made and an Islamic tradition of nursing began. Arab ideas were later influential in Europe. The famous Knights Hospitaller arose as a group of individuals associated with an Amalfitan hospital in Jerusalem, which was built to provide care for poor, sick or injured Christian pilgrims to the Holy Land. Following the capture of the city by Crusaders, the order became a military as well as infirmarian order.

Roman Catholic orders such as the Franciscans stressed tending the sick, especially during the devastating plague.

https://www.newadvent.org/cathen/07477a.htm

# REFERENCES

De Witt (2009). *Fundamental Concepts and Skills for Nursing.* Missouri: Saunders Elsevier.

Dock, L, & Nutting, A. (1917). *A History of Nursing: the evolution of nursing systems from the earliest times to the foundation for the first English and American training school for Nurses.* New York: G.P Putnam.

Helmstadter, C., & Groden, J. (2016). *Nursing before Nightingale 1815-1899.* London: Routledge.

Jones, C. (1989). *The Charitable Imperative. Hospitals and Nursing in Ancient Regimé and Revolutionary France.* London: Routledge.

Mc Gregor-Robertson, J. (1902). *The Household Physician.* London: Gresham Publishing.

Miller-Rosser., Chapman, Y., & Francis, K. (2009). *Historical, Cultural, and Contemporary Influences on the Status of Women in Nursing in Saudi Arabia.* Online Journal of Issues in Nursing, 11, 1-15.

Orey, M. (2010). *Emerging perspectives on Learning, Teaching and Technology.* North Charleston: Create Space.

Staggers, N. (2008). Nanotechnology: The coming revolution and its implications for consumers, clinicians and informatics. Nursing Outlook Sep-Oct;56(5):268-74. doi: 10.1016/j.outlook.2008.06.004.

Stewart, I. & Austin, A. (1962). *A History of Nursing from Ancient to Modern Times.* N.Y.: Putnam Books.

Zhang, R., Burgess, E., Rothrock, N., Rasmussen, L., Batt, S., Butt., Z. (2019). Provider perspectives on the integration of patient reported outcomes in an electronic health record. Journal of the American Medical Informatics Association. April 2(1): 73-80.

www.ingramcontent.com/pod-product-compliance
Lightning Source LLC
Chambersburg PA
CBHW060617200326
41521CB00007B/798